Gulf War Nurses

Gulf War Nurses

*Personal Accounts of 14 Americans,
1990–1991 and 2003–2010*

edited by PATRICIA RUSHTON

McFarland & Company, Inc., Publishers
Jefferson, North Carolina, and London

The interview with Susan Herron Thompson originally appeared in P. Rushton, L.C. Callister, and M. Wilson, *Latter-day Saint Nurses at War: A Story of Caring and Sacrifice* (Provo, Utah: Religious Studies Center, Brigham Young University, 2005), 209–223. Reprinted with permission.

LIBRARY OF CONGRESS CATALOGUING-IN-PUBLICATION DATA

Gulf War nurses : personal accounts of 14 Americans, 1990–1991 and 2003–2010 / edited by Patricia Rushton.
     p.   cm.
    Includes bibliographical references and index.

    ISBN 978-0-7864-6073-1
    softcover : 50# alkaline paper ∞

    1. United States—Armed Forces—Nurses—Biography. 2. Persian Gulf War, 1991—Medical care. 3. Persian Gulf War, 1991—Personal narratives, American. 4. Iraq War, 2003—Medical care—United States. 5. Iraq War, 2003—Personal narratives, American. I. Rushton, Patricia.
UH493.G85   2011
956.7044'27—dc22   2010043214
[B]

British Library cataloguing data are available

Front cover: Camp Hospital in Balad, Iraq; *from left* U.S. Navy, Air Force and Army nursing insignia

Manufactured in the United States of America

McFarland & Company, Inc., Publishers
  Box 611, Jefferson, North Carolina 28640
  www.mcfarlandpub.com

TABLE OF CONTENTS

INTRODUCTION

It would seem that those who benefit the most from nursing care, the patients and their families, have little real understanding of what it means to be "a nurse." Some have said to this editor that nurses never lead, but only follow. They never make decisions, but only obey the command of others. Yet in all my years as a nurse, I have seen my colleagues make important decisions and take actions that saved patients discomfort, misery, and their lives. I have interviewed nurses for the Nurses at War project whose decisions have made profound differences in nursing practice and patient care. Though the following accounts only embrace the experiences of a few nurses who served during the conflicts in the Persian Gulf during the late twentieth and early twenty-first centuries, I wish to assure the reader that nurses in every war have made important decisions that have great impact on themselves, their colleagues, and most importantly, their patients and families.

On August 2, 1990, Iraq invaded Kuwait, a nation friendly to the United States. For some citizens of the United States, this event may have been too far away and too disconnected from daily life to have been noteworthy. Some of us, however, did look up and take note. The United States had not been in an active, declared "war" type of conflict since the Vietnam War. But I and some of my nursing colleagues associated with military reserve units realized that the invasion of Kuwait could turn into something warmer than a political conversation between two nations.

I joined the military reserve as a member of the United States Navy Nurse Corps reserve in 1967. I had been active reserve in the United States Navy Nurse Corps, stationed at the Philadelphia Naval Hospital during the Vietnam War. At the end of my three-year active duty obligation at that hospital, I remained a drilling Nurse Corps reservist, drilling one weekend a month and two weeks a year. I understood that the reason the Navy was paying me to drill was so that I would be prepared to go to war if necessary. Now, it appeared, there could be a war and there was a very good probability that I and some of my friends and professional colleagues would be recalled and mobilized. We began to make plans.

I and a nursing associate went to the nursing administrator at the hospital in which we worked and explained there was a possibility we could be recalled to active duty for the potential conflict between Kuwait and Iraq. We also noted that a high percentage of the nursing staff in that facility were associated with the several military reserve units. If all were recalled, there could be a serious dent in the hospital's nursing staff. The administrator was a bit incredulous that this might happen.

I began to make an effort to complete projects at work and to find people who could fill in if necessary. I made those I worked with aware of the possibility of mobilization. They were also disbelieving of the situation. One work associate said, "If they send you orders, you are actually going to go?" as if I had a physical or moral choice. My response was, "Well, after this many years, it is a little late to tell them no. That's what they have been paying me for."

My mother was suffering from a terminal illness. Her response to my news that I may have to go away from home was: "You can't leave 'til I die." I knew her remaining life would not be long, and I prayed that I would not have to go until she no longer needed me at her side. In this way I was fortunate and not mobilized until about a month after she passed away.

The "shock and awe" of a real-life wartime situation was overwhelming for so many. Nonmilitary citizens had a hard time connecting with the idea of fighting an actual war. Even for those of us who knew it could be a possibility, the reality of it was stunning. An associate was called the week before Memorial Day and told to be at her duty station, two states away, by the Sunday before Memorial Day. She had forty-eight hours to prepare before actually leaving her home and driving to her mobilization site. Some were surprised when they arrived at their mobilization destinations to find out they probably wouldn't have weekends, nights, or holidays free as they had in their civilian situations. Some found themselves working in areas in which they had little expertise; i.e., the psychiatric or operating room nurse who ended up working on a general medical-surgical unit. One nurse had changed her career path and was working in a government civil service area while maintaining her activity in a reserve medical unit. She was mobilized to be the chief nursing officer at a major military medical center. All of us were distressed and frustrated by the lack of information available to us about the developing situation, as decisions were made far above our pay grade and took awhile to trickle down. Active duty nurses were called up by their unit supervisors, told to pack their gear and be at a pickup site within a few days or hours to be mobilized to forward positions such as hospital ships or medical centers in Europe or on the battle front in the Middle East.

Members of active and reserve military medical units just picked themselves up, prepared and went. They coped with whatever situation they found themselves in, trying to do their tasks in the best way they could. In many situations their previous experiences helped them make changes at their mobilization sites that maintained and improved the efficiency in which patient care was provided. They sacrificed for each other. One nurse was responsible for making assignments that would send her colleagues into harm's way. At one point she realized how much her colleagues had already given and asked to go herself before having to send someone to the Gulf on a second tour. Nurses in the Gulf managed their work schedules to allow associates to have badly needed downtime. Nurses who remained in the United States at military health care facilities felt they were sacrificing the "better part" so that their colleagues could go to the battle front. They did not realize what a difference they would make in the lives of military members and their families stationed in the States during the conflict.

The nurses during the Gulf War conflicts have all done "what they had to do." In the several years I have been collecting the accounts of nurses who have served during wartime, I have never had a nurse come to me and say, "I have this great, heroic story to tell you." They all say, "I didn't do anything special. I just did what I had to do." Yet, because they did "what they had to do," they were heroic. They served their country, acknowledging their commitment to the principles of freedom for which this country stands. They took care of patients and families, making decisions that made a difference in the quality of life and death. They were often the individuals making the top-level decisions that influenced troop movements and patient care. They endured to the end, usually without recognition or reward for their actions. They came home to apply the lessons they learned from their military experience to the care of their civilian patients, their civilian positions and often to their own families.

It is hoped that the stories told in here will serve several purposes. These stories acknowledge the amazing work of the individuals who have shared their experiences. They highlight the essential work of military nurses specifically, and the nursing profession in general. Finally, the accounts provide lessons of commitment, hard work, creativity, service and honor from which all can learn.

The Nurses at War Project

Since the work of Florence Nightingale, Dorothea Dix, and Clara Barton, professional nurses have been involved in caring for the sick and wounded during military conflicts. The collection of these accounts is of great benefit to nurse historians and others studying those who have served during military conflicts. Collecting and archiving these accounts is critical because most of the nurses who served in World War I have died and nurses who served during World War II are now in their eighties, some with fading memories and declining health. Many voices are lost each day as this generation passes.

The Nurses at War project is a continuing long-term project to gather the accounts of nurses who have served during wartime. Accounts are gathered from nurses willing to tell their stories regardless of the war, the branch of military service, the site of service or the type of nursing performed by the participant. The main goal of the project is to acquire the accounts and experiences while the nurses are able to relate them. A second goal is to share these accounts, in some way, through presentation and publication.

Several common themes emerged as nurses discussed both their professional and personal experiences. The main theme was: "We did what we had to do." They had chosen a profession that required their very best in physical strength and intellectual creativity. Professional themes included short staffing, long hours, and insufficient supplies calling for creativity and ingenuity in clinical practice.

Nurses treated victims of shock and trauma, as many of them practiced before the establishment of critical care units in the 1960s. They cared for patients with post–traumatic stress syndrome, which was not identified as an official diagnosis until after the Vietnam War. They cared for patients with unusual diseases not typically seen in clinical practice, including jungle rot and other skin conditions typical in the Pacific theater in World War II. Sometimes they were in situations that required to provide care beyond their scope of practice under very difficult circumstances. Often they had profound emotional experiences.

Some study participants made meaning of their wartime experiences and described the lessons learned that profoundly affected their lives. These included living fully in the present, reevaluating priorities, cherishing freedom, valuing home and family, and having faith and trust in God. These were the values they held fast to and which sustained them in difficult times. Study participants are very patriotic and speak of cherishing freedom, even in those instances where they had conflicting feelings about going to war. Valuing home and family is a pervasive theme in the interviews and in the letters written home. These nurses espoused a spiritual lifestyle, and this is a common thread throughout the interviews. They found strength in their relationship with a higher power and made meaning of their experiences because of their religious beliefs.

On November 11, 2004, Veterans Day, a note dedicated to nurses was left at the Vietnam War Memorial. It read, "I don't remember your name, but thanks for saving my life." This indication of how much the quiet, unsung, heroic services of a nurse meant to this veteran is inspiring. These men and women have made a difference in the lives of countless military personnel — and though the patients may not remember their names, they remember the quiet presence and dedicated and competent care they received from a nurse.

PATRICK AMERSBACH

The experience of Patrick Amersbach during the Persian Gulf War demonstrates the versatility and flexibility of military nurses during a time of war. As good nurses do, military nurses learn with each new experience and use that knowledge to make decisions about good patient care. Besides his Navy experience, Patrick started out as an Army enlisted man, working his way up through the enlisted ranks. He chose to leave the Army, go to school and come back into the Navy. He tells his wartime experience.

My first assignment was Naval Hospital Bremerton, Washington. Bremerton is a medium-sized military treatment facility with the inpatient general medicine bed capability of less than 100. I initially went to the medical-orthopedic floor and learned my basic nursing and medical-surgical skills there. Most medical-surgical units are a good place to start due to their variety of patient populations. On that particular unit you could be exposed to adults or geriatrics with multiple medical problems or fresh post–operative patients. You could have an 80-year-old with congestive heart failure or an 18-year-old who broke a wrist from falling off a skateboard.

After about a year and a half on the medical-orthopedic ward, I was transferred to the intensive care unit (ICU) for a short period of time. I was like most people, at least in Navy nursing. We seem to have an idea of what we want to do within the profession — a goal, more or less. On the unit I'm currently privileged to lead, I have 25 ensigns and lieutenant junior grade Nurse Corps officers, and of them 16 to 18 know exactly where they want to head in nursing, at least their short-term goals. Again, I was no different than them at that point in my career. I spent just enough time in the intensive care unit to give me a working knowledge of the complexities of the critical care patient before taking over a small outpatient clinic. My total time in Bremerton was about three and a half years before moving to the Administrative Support Unit (ASU) in Manama, Bahrain.

I was stationed in Bahrain for a one year unaccompanied isolated tour from January 1998 to January 1999. Bahrain is an island nation about 11 miles off the coast of Saudi Arabia. Its significance was a result of a growing U.S. presence in the Persian Gulf after the Gulf War in 1990–1991. It was a great tour. I actually asked for it. I wanted to be somewhere close to where the action

5

was, because as far as I'm concerned that's why I wear a uniform. I was supposed to go to the USS *Theodore Roosevelt* as the ship's nurse. When I was up for orders, they were putting junior lieutenants aboard. When I was supposed to actually receive my orders to the ship, they changed the requirements, stating now that they wanted more senior lieutenants and lieutenant commanders aboard. I was in contact with a detailer at the time. She was apologetic, which was nice. She said she'd keep me in mind for anything else that popped up. Being a little bit older and more mature, I knew what billets were available. I requested assignment to the Middle East. I went to Bahrain as a junior lieutenant although the skill set for junior Nurse Corps officers isn't usually enough to be a benefit to anyone over there.

By the time I got there in 1998, it was a fixed installation that provided support to the Navy Central Command (NAVCENT) and the Fifth Fleet, including ships and battle groups that entered the Persian Gulf. The medical department of the ASU was billeted for two Nurse Corps officers, but when I walked in the door, no one had been at my position for three months. The desk had cobwebs and a stack full of old manuals and assorted junk. The office and its contents had been pilfered for things that were of real use. The medical department's mission was to provide direct medical support to the fleet or battle groups and coordinate more definitive care if required. I was the liaison to the civilian hospitals in Manama, the capitol of Bahrain. It sounds scary until you get out there and realize how international the population is. Bahrain isn't going to be oil rich for as long as many of the other Persian Gulf nations. It has a large and very international banking community. If I remember correctly, it has the largest aluminum smelting plants in that part of the world. It also has an increasingly productive ship building capability. They're looking beyond their oil to survive.

In addition to outpatient medical care, an example of what we did there would be to address the needs of a sailor that requires medical attention greater than could be provided aboard the ship. Almost all of them would come through our medical department prior to being placed in one of the surrounding hospitals. I guess you could say we were the gatekeepers and would determine whether or not their care could be taken care of locally or if, in fact, they needed to be medically evacuated (medevac) back to the United States. As you could imagine, it could be very scary for a service member to be in a Bahraini hospital by themselves. We did everything we could to keep tabs on them and put their fears to rest. The hospitals were very safe and clean, and most of the medical staff was U.S. or British trained. Nursing staff predominantly came out of India, the Philippines, Pakistan, Ireland, or England, so communication wasn't really an issue. Every day we helped someone out at the Salmaniya Medical Center, International Hospital of Bahrain or American Mission Hospital. If nothing else, just showing our face, shaking hands and spreading goodwill to our servicemen and women in those hospitals made a big difference for them. As I mentioned before, it was a great tour. I got to see, do, and participate in everything I could possibly get myself into—from being launched off the deck of an aircraft carrier after completing their "in-theater medical briefs" to attending embassy parties to a humanitarian recovery mission off the coast of Somalia.

The recovery mission was unique. Out of the blue one morning my department head asked me if I had any experience with human remains. I said, "Sure. I'm a nurse." Up to that point my experience had been very limited in the intensive care unit or on a medical-surgical ward. I was thinking, "How hard could it be?" Shortly after that a team was assembled and we were off flying over Saudi Arabia. The team comprised a medical team and SPRINT team. A SPRINT team is a mental health team used to help those that had been exposed to a traumatic event. In this situation a Somali ferry with about a 180 people capsized. The afternoon we arrived, a U.S. Naval ship, the USNS Saturn, was transiting the Red Sea area when one of the lookouts saw the bodies from the ferry floating around. They stopped the ship right there, called for assistance, and began the process of recovering the bodies.

The United Nations was involved and more or less took care of us. We were flown down by a Navy transport and landed in Yemen. The airport had only half of its runway lights working. There was no radar and there were burnt-out tanks on the side of the runway. It was very concerning for the pilots and aircrew. We had to stay in Yemen overnight at a local hotel. That was interesting. It had barbed wire all around it, and it appeared to be the only building in the area that had electricity. There was a civil war there years before. I believe the city of Aden, where we were, was the capital. The next morning the UN got us back out to the airfield where the helicopters off of the USNS Saturn picked us up and flew us out to the ship so we could deal with the bodies.

Of the 180 people on board, there were 33 bodies recovered with no way to identify what was left. They don't have dental records, DNA, or stuff like that to track them like we do. The condition of the bodies went from advanced decomposition to just parts of bodies. We couldn't do much other than put them in bodybags and bury them at sea. The UN flew a couple of Islamic clergymen on board the ship to pray over the remains in accordance with their beliefs. We separated the men from the women, if we could tell the difference, and had the heads facing east. We tried to do what was right for them in accordance with the clergymen's directions. Once that was done, we lowered the bodies back into the sea, one or two at a time. Overall it involved an aircrew and aircraft, four officers and four corpsmen from Bahrain, and the crew of the ship. It was a lot of people for something that wasn't really our affair. After that we stayed with the ship and sailed back to Bahrain.

One of the more enjoyable parts of the job in Bahrain was flying out to the carrier battle groups to give the in-theater briefs to the medical departments. This included telling them what capabilities we had there in Bahrain in order to support the fleet, what the local hospitals could do, and if necessary, what we needed to do to set up medevacs.

The tour was a huge exposure to a new culture, a new religion for me, and a very dynamic and a very open society for a Persian Gulf nation. I was there for a year, from 1998 to 1999. Then I went to Oak Harbor, Washington.

Oak Harbor is on Whidbey Island, north of Seattle. Bremerton is across the Puget Sound from Seattle. It looks pretty close on a map, but in reality, it's a one-lane highway with numerous travel inconveniences. However, it was a great place for kids—roads are safe, nice green environment. There are bad influences everywhere you go, but truly these are minimized up there. I was there for almost four years. While I was there I worked at a multipurpose ward for almost a year. That means you walk in the door and you take care of a six-year-old asthmatic with their breathing treatments, a 56-year-old in for chest pain, and the woman in the labor and delivery room who is delivering. You have to go back and take care of the newborn, assess them, do the APGAR scores and ensure the baby is safe and healthy. I had not done that type of nursing before—babies? Are you kidding me? It's not my favorite, but you thrive where you're planted and you do what you're supposed to and you do the best you can. Really it was a good experience. Navy nursing tries to keep relatively experienced nurses in those remote areas because of the variety of patients that you have—21-year-old active-duty sailors, post–operative patients, medicine and pediatric all rolled into one unit. It says a lot about the skill set of a Navy nurse.

From there, I went to ambulatory care environment and was a clinic nurse assigned to nine providers—two flight surgeons, two physician assistants, and five family practice physicians. That was also a different type of nursing. From there I went to staff education for the last portion of my time there. I did training for newly assigned staff and basic, advanced, and pediatric training for the command.

After Oak Harbor, I had orders to San Diego Naval Hospital. Prior to reporting to the command, I got a call from the nurse placement officer. Initially I was supposed to go to ER. Then they called and said, "Hey, we've got a job for you." I was like, "Oh nice." Usually when they call you to offer you a job, it's a job nobody else wants. As it turned out, it was a captain I had worked with when I was an ensign in Washington. She said, "I remember you. I have a job for you as a division officer."

I came to San Diego, checked in and took over as division officer of a medical-surgical area. My friend, the captain, said, "Well, I was thinking you'd be great. It's a lot of responsibility. It's a leadership position, and you have the required skill set and a demeanor to handle such a position." They were half flattering and half pushing, so I took it, and I haven't regretted it. After my Iraq duty, I am back in San Diego with a staff of about 60, with about a dozen brand new nurses. I have about 31 nurses overall and between 30 and 36 corpsmen, depending on the day of the week and the rotation. They all spend some time on the floor, usually a year or two, get their initial training in the inpatient setting, then move on to someplace else within the command. It's a lot of staff, and leadership is a privilege at any level. I'm a naval officer first, and then a nurse; and I take it seriously, but also enjoy it.

It's a departure from many nurses, and I think it has a lot to do with the culture I grew up with in the military; wearing camouflage, carrying a rifle and being a staff sergeant, pushing troops, being a platoon sergeant. You understand the foundation of leadership is order and discipline, which are important at all levels. I had my initial military training. Then I earned my nursing degree, unlike most folks who do it the other way around. It can be hard to figure out both at the same time. I'm responsible for helping the nurses balance the two, and often it's very difficult.

We have a great relationship between most of the units. We have clinical nurse specialists (CNS) that are master's prepared and are the experts in the medical-surgical environment, understanding the clinical issues. When staffing allows, you also have your division officer for administrative issues on each unit. I can focus on addressing military issues, professional issues, administrative issues, counseling issues, all those other things that many times get pushed aside because they're not as important as taking care of the patients. Many wouldn't want the job of a division officer on such a busy unit with little to no clinical time and a lot of responsibility. Even for me, any day of the week it can be painful, causing you to pull your hair out, but it all boils down to the fact that leadership is a privilege. I've had the opportunity to teach and to mentor very junior Nurse Corps officers and help them develop as naval officers. If they decide to stay in, great. If they don't, they can look back on it and say, "I can understand and see why that perspective was taken or why he did the things the way he did."

I arrived at the hospital at the end of July 2003 and got turned over to the Marines for deployment to Iraq in January 2004. I was there for seven months. I had just figured out how to come in the door at the hospital and off to Iraq I went. I was assigned to Alpha Surgical Company or 1st Medical Battalion. I stood on the desk to volunteer to be deployed. It's not that I wanted to get out of my position. It's a very important position, and I knew in some respects I would be "kneecapping" my ward. I had already started to implement things, making changes and now I'm gone. One of the reasons I came to San Diego from Oak Harbor was to get to an operational platform. Oak Harbor is so small they don't have any operations billets assigned to them for a general nurse. It was important for me. I could have been assigned to a smaller facility and run into the same issue. I wear a uniform to support and defend the needs of our nation as directed by chief of naval operations and the National Security Council, and everybody else. That's my job. I wanted to support the Marines in the field. I knew there was an upcoming rotation, and when it was time to support that, I made sure I was lined up to be one of the top people on the list, and it worked.

I can't say I went strictly clinical because I was the officer in charge of the ward and evacuation platoon for Alpha Surgical Company. Other than the nurse anesthetist (CRNA), I was the senior nurse, but that's not saying much when there's only three of you assigned. I was also the force protection officer, so I had to make sure that the structures were hardened, sand bagged, and instruct the chain of command on how to protect the physical facilities in the event of a rocket or mortar attack, or indirect or direct fire. It's odd for a nurse, but it came from my seven years as military police and the physical security operations that I was familiar with and had an interest in. I also had between nine and twelve corpsmen assigned and we ran seven months of medical coverage for the wounded and casualties that came through our surgical company.

You name it, we saw it. It's funny because I've got some of the e-mails I sent back to my family after our first rocket attack, after our first casualties, my first medevac flight — bagging a patient for 45 minutes, 150 to 500 feet off the deck at 120 knots. Some of it's humorous and some of it is dead serious.

We were staged in Kuwait for about three weeks waiting to move forward. Transportation was always an issue. You get antsy. You feel like your training is inadequate for what you're going to be facing. Alpha Surgical Company was broken up in Kuwait. We were stripped of our general and orthopedic surgeon. We showed up in Iraq with a less than optimal unit, and we were expected to do the best we can, and of course we did. That's how we started out.

We landed out there and took over for the Army. The Army staff said it was a very safe place. You don't have to worry about anything. There hasn't been anything going on here since the beginning of the war. The Army left and three days later we got hit with Chinese-made 122 millimeter rockets that were being bracketed across what we call our downtown area where our troops were being housed. One died instantly, another one died of his wounds in Germany, and two more were wounded 50 meters to 70 meters from our surgical company.

We had sporadic rocket attacks and other little incursion issues throughout our stay, many of the rockets hitting the downtown area. Fortunately the Yugoslavian's built the base, so most of their structures were capable of withstanding small fragments from the munitions. I was out in Al Asad, located in the Anbar Province. It was a captured Iraqi air base built back in 1987 by the Yugoslavians. It had huge runways and could handle any aircraft in our Air Force inventory, and as a result it was a major supply point for that region. We were fortunate that we had that kind of support if we needed it.

The first rocket attack was within a week of the Army pulling out. The first casualties showed up the first day that we were getting our medical equipment. We're all off-loading our medical equipment and the first CH-53 lands and we get our first really bad patients. I had to look back at my e-mails to see how many there were and what their dispositions were. I e-mailed my family as often as I could. Initially our computer access was a bit sketchy, so you would write and write and write and when you got a chance to mail it out, you would mail it out. Again, with it being such a big base and actually belonging to the Third Marine Air Wing (3rdMAW), they had the infrastructure, personnel and equipment to outfit the place very well, although it took some time to take over for the Army and change the systems. After the transition we were able to e-mail very frequently.

It was hit and miss with casualties. I'll give you the numbers— 400 wounded in action, and something ridiculous like 4000–6000 patient contacts from non–battle disease and injuries. The non–battle disease and injuries constituted a lot of what we did. With the first battle of Fallujah, we picked up a lot of casualties. We were also getting them from the Syrian border and all over from western Iraq. We were the big hub, more or less. They would come from the small FRSSs, or the resuscitative units. We're supposed to retriage and treat them if we can, stabilize them if required, and put them in another helicopter and send them out if critical.

The helicopters can't transit from the Syrian border all the way to Baghdad, which was a level three facility that had a CT scanner, neurosurgery, and all of the specialists seen in a trauma hospital. Alpha Surgical Company was a level two unit. Level one is a basic hospital corpsmen or medic at the aid station or in the field right next to the infantry Marine or soldier. Level two has some basic surgical capability and a reduced pharmacy; but may not have lab or X-ray capability; but because they have a surgeon they're a level two. My surgical company is the same as an FRSS with the exception that we have X-ray capability, a larger pharmacy, and a very basic lab capability. Level three is a combat support hospital, or at least that's what the Army calls them. The Navy calls them fleet hospitals or expeditionary units now, which have CT scanners, a plethora of specialty surgeons and ICUs. We wouldn't have an ICU at level two, although they said we did. We had impact ventilators, little tiny ventilators, and that was about it, with larger O2 tanks to support that. So that's a level one, two, and three facility. Level four would be Germany, overseas, or basically any stateside military treatment facility.

We saw it all: scorpion bites, cellulitis, orthopedic injuries and combat wounded. Marines get bored from time to time, and they would find them-

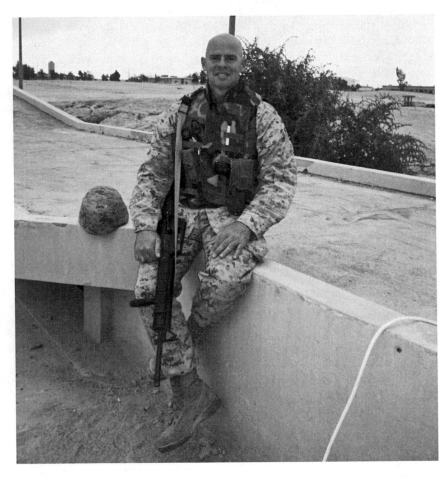

Patrick Amersbach the morning after an attack. In past wars, nurses have not been issued weapons. In this war and depending on the unit assigned, they did carry weapons and were trained to use them.

selves playing with spiders or other critters. One unique type is the camel spider. They can run up to 30 miles per hour and can jump three feet. They like to stay in the shadows and will run away from sunlight. It keeps you up at night a little bit.

We had superb mental health services out there, whether it was the psych technicians or the actual psychiatrists. It was good because it kept a lot of those who required services out in the field, engaged in what they were doing and focused, versus sending them to the rear for treatment or evaluation. As a result of the mental health services being at the front, they were able to very quickly determine if some of these people needed to get out of there quickly.

I believe it was born out of Desert Storm. I know the Army went to great lengths to insure that they had psychologists at the battalion level, so they were responsible to address the needs of anywhere from 250 to 400 troops. Whether or not it was successful in every unit, I don't even know. It's something that started in that time frame, and continued with OIF and OEF.

There were a lot of patients that came through our surgical company. One jumped on grenades to save his buddies. I think some of the emotional difficulties had a lot do to with the inexperience of the staff that was out there. Of my two nurses, the first one had about a year of experience in the Navy and as a nurse. The other nurse had almost two years of experience prior to being deployed out there. Even for the physicians, combat trauma is different than going to the OR to work on a patient. Combat trauma is a lot different than taking care of patients aboard a ship. Most situations usually include a clean, sterile environment, with most accidents industrial in nature, verses a traumatic injury resulting from an explosion or bullet.

The patient who jumped on a grenade to save his buddy came in during a period of increased casualties. He was put off to the side as an expectant, a patient that was expected to die. Then he started showing some signs of survival and was retriaged and immediately flown out. We had close to a dozen casualties come in at the same time with limited resources, so you really have to take a look at who your patients are and what triage category would be appropriate for them. It's not an easy decision. He was quickly medevaced to Frankfurt, then on to Walter Reed where his family was able to meet up with him prior to his dying from his wounds.

Then there are the funny ones, and there's a lot to be said about humor in very stressful situations. I had this one corpsman who took a piece of shrapnel in his butt. He and his two other buddies came in by helicopter after hitting a roadside bomb. He was big! I mean he was fluffy. I had to carry him on the stretcher so I just cussed at him the whole time, and he just laughed and laughed. He just had a little piece of shrapnel in his butt; it was one of those million dollar wounds. I thought, "You've got to be kidding. This is killing me! He's got to be 250 pounds and I'm carrying him." I have no idea how he got to the Gulf.

Another was a 21-year-old that had a year and a half of college before going into the Marines. He was an infantryman who was assigned up in the machine-gun ring of a Humvee. His training didn't include engaging the enemy behind a machine gun in a moving vehicle. They were ambushed and his first instinct was to duck below the shield of the gun instead of returning fire. Bullets are whizzing through the vehicle and he takes one in the leg. He couldn't bring himself up to the gun to return fire because of the heavy volume of fire, lack of training, and possibly fear — not that he could have done anything at that point anyway. He was going to have adjustment issues when he

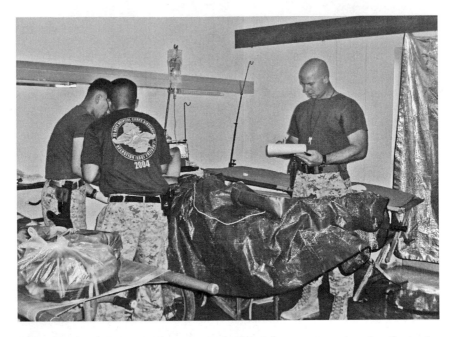

Every day the corpsmen and nurses worked together as a team to get patients stabilized for surgery or transport, if that was the next step. Patrick Amersbach (right) and two corpsmen are assessing and treating a foreign national who was wounded as he ran through a checkpoint on one of the main supply routes near the base.

left the theater because he felt like he had let his team down, with numerous Marines in his unit being wounded. Again he was young, inexperienced and was doing something that he wasn't trained for. Basically, infantrymen are trained to cover, return fire, rush to the objective cover, and return fire. He covered, but never got an opportunity to return fire, so he had guilt associated with that. I spent hours talking to him. He was afraid that he was going to disappoint his father, let the Marines down, the whole nine yards.

We got report of six casualties coming in. These kids, and they are kids, arrived in the back of a seven-ton truck. There were only four of them, not half a dozen, and they've all got shrapnel wounds. An improvised explosive device blew up their Humvee. They're so peppered we couldn't count the number of shrapnel wounds — shrapnel, dirt, rock debris, the rest of it. We had to dispense morphine to these kids like it was going out of style, 10–15 milligrams at a time, as you're picking out the pieces that you can.

We cared for some local folk. One Iraqi and two Egyptians who decided to run a checkpoint were engaged by the troops at the checkpoint. They got bullet wounds and fragments in their backs because they ran their truck through the checkpoint and the guards opened up on them. Not too smart.

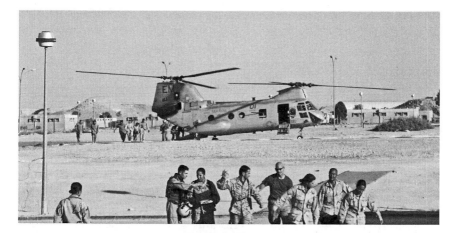

The CH-46 Sea Knight, sometimes known as the "frog," was designed primarily as an all-conditions, assault transport for combat Marines, supplies, and equipment during amphibious and subsequent operations ashore. It normally has a crew of four or five and can carry up to 14 litters with two additional medical attendants onboard. This level two surgical company depended on them and other rotary aircraft to bring the combat wounded in for treatment as well as to the combat support hospitals in Balad or Baghdad for more advanced care if required. Patrick Amersbach and others are receiving casualties from an unknown location in western Iraq. Pictured are members of the Navy, Marines, and the Army, highlighting the close working relationship from all services and the importance of interoperability in a combat zone.

There was also a ten-year-old girl with a congenital heart condition we were taking care of. Basically, we ended up being her primary care managers. How this girl got on the base every time she needed care was amazing, but she did. It was one of those cases that was going to be turned over to the state department for a possible adoption by a hospital system to perform the surgery, but I don't know what happened with that. There are a lot of them like that.

There are all kind of patients. Only a certain portion we dealt with were actually combat wounds. There were a lot more mental issues that needed a little bit of addressing and tweaking, than medical issues. Kidney stones caused by dehydration were very common. It was amazing how many we saw. There was actually a kid out there who had one kidney removed prior to coming into the Marines, was on active duty, and now he's in a hot, dry combat zone with one kidney. I don't remember what we were seeing him for, if it was symptoms of kidney stones or what, but he had to be sent back to the States. I don't know if he donated to his brother or what. He shouldn't have been in the Marines in the first place.

I had to transport a patient at three o' clock in the morning, 150 to 500 feet off the ground, at night, with a gunship escort out to one of the combat support hospitals in Balad, and he was dead. I was ventilating the patient for 55 minutes, trying to do an epinephrine drip, with no pump, with no way to determine what would be an appropriate dose, just trying everything I can to keep this guy's heart going until we get to more definitive care. It was dark, no lights, and blackout conditions. I had a monitor attached to him, but a monitor is only good in stable conditions. Aircraft are not stable. The wave forms were crappy. There was no blood pressure. There was a pulse, but who knows how real that was. I sure didn't know. So we pull him off the helicopter, roll him in, and the Army doctor asks, "How long has he been this way?" I said, "The whole way over." The doctor says, "He's dead." It was tragic. My 55 minutes of bagging a patient doesn't really mean anything. We had to try, but if he was dead when I got him aboard the helicopter, then it just means that four more lives were at risk. I was stuck in Balad.

The sirens went off, and the sirens only go off after the rockets impact. Makes sense, doesn't it? I was scurrying around doing what I could to find any flights to get out of there to get back to Al Asad for two reasons: One, I don't like rocket or mortar attacks. They get a little old after a while. And two, I had left my two junior nurses by themselves. They were telling me it would be another day or so before I could fly back. No way! I could find a flight. I could do that and I did.

I hooked up with some guys with vodka and cigarettes, and we talked the Russians into flying us back. The Russian pilot was unshaven for four or five days, wearing cut-off shorts, a tank top T-shirt, and flip-flops, with a cigarette and a cup of tea in his hand and a look about him that reminded me of someone that shouldn't be trusted to drive a cab, let alone fly a four-engine jet transport. I got on the plane and laundry was hanging from the hydraulic lines. There's a huge cardboard cut-out of Santa Claus and Rudolph taped to the inside. That bothered me a little bit more, but not so much that I wanted to hang out at the air base anymore. It was like an old movie. It was like *Kelly's Heroes* or something that had Clint Eastwood in it. This old tank driver was played by Donald Sutherland, kind of a hippie, free spirit kind of guy. That was my pilot. That will all stay with me for a long while.

The things that were painful per se, they go away. It's the funny things or the first time or the unique things that stay with me — my first flight taking a patient out with a good patient outcome. That's good, always good. Flying back and watching red tracers coming up at the helicopter — yeah, that's kind of neat, great firework show. You land and the crew gets out and the whole crew runs their hands all along the skin of the helicopter looking for holes. I haven't had to do that before. Next flight coming back, the Marine attack helicopter picked up on something on its night sensors because it starts firing its three-barrel, 20-millimeter cannon at the target. I'm watching the tracers go off. It was nice for a change. It's hot and muggy, you are sweating through

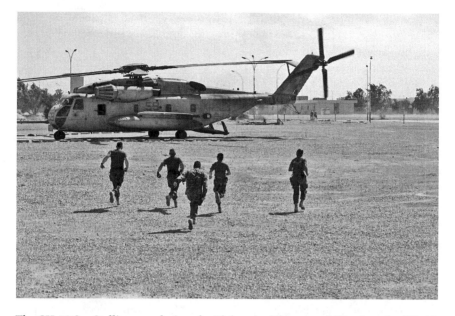

The CH-53 Sea Stallion was designed with heavier lifting capability than the CH-46, making it suitable for assault transport, aircraft recovery, personnel transport, and medical evacuation. The helicopter seats 37 passengers in its normal configuration, with provisions to carry 55 passengers with centerline seats installed, or up to 24 litter patients. With its dual-point hook system, it can carry external loads of up to 26,000 pounds. It has a crew of four to six and is armed with two M240 or M2 machine guns. Patrick Amersbach and his fellow soldiers are running out to a CH-53E that just landed from an unknown destination. Due to lapses in communications they often did not know the number or the severity of the casualties until the aircraft landed.

your clothes the entire flight. Helicopters aren't air-conditioned, and it doesn't matter if it's at night, it's still 100 degrees, beating at you at a 100 miles per hour. They're things that I'll never forget. To say that I enjoyed it sounds kind of awful, but I did enjoy it. It's what I wear a uniform for. I would go back, although I may not get that offer. The command here has gone to a tiered program. If you've been deployed basically greater than 180 days then you're not eligible. There are plenty of people who haven't done that yet, so unless you have a very specific skill set, you don't go back. I was there 240 days, or about eight months.

Towards the end of our deployment they moved in a squadron of Marine attack aircraft, which is always nice to have. They stayed and I believe are still there. It's good because it saves the department of defense a lot of money. If you think about it, taking a carrier battle group into the Persian Gulf and letting them do circles up there in the Gulf while the air groups conduct operations to support ground forces is awfully expensive. If you can take a squadron and put them on the ground there, at least you don't have to expend fuel and the rest of what is required for the ships to float in the Gulf. We had helicopter support, an Army air ambulance unit who did 90 percent of our medevacs. They were a great asset to have and worked very well with us.

My family did okay while I was gone. I kept in contact through e-mails. I have two sons. One is in the Coast Guard Academy located at New London, Connecticut. The other one was at Washington State University. They're older. They're not little kids. They knew what was going on. I was on the phone talking to my wife at the time a rocket attack occurred. You could hear the impacts, and I said, "Gotta go, gotta go," then clink, hung the phone up. That was a bit disconcerting for her. As long as you can call back within a reasonable amount of time, the freak-out factor isn't as great.

I did whatever I could while I was there, and not just from a nursing perspective, but from a military perspective — Like the force protection responsibilities, making sure that the buildings are sandbagged and hardened. When we first got there the philosophy of the unit commander was that we needed to go to the bunker every time we got intelligence that we may be attacked. That means you need to leave your barracks or leave the surgical company and go to a bunker. A Chinese-made 122 rocket fired from a piece of PVC pipe from a range of about 12 miles is not going to penetrate the roof of these buildings because they're semihardened. Chinese 107 and 122 mm rockets are antipersonnel with a lot of little fragments designed to kill people in the open and not armor-piercing or something that's supposed to penetrate through a hardened shelter or bunker. Basically it's like a bottle rocket. They would fire it and they would hope to hit something. It's not like they had sophisticated rocket launchers. They were very ingenious rocket launchers, and they could bury them or they could leave them where they were, it didn't make a difference. We had impacts directly on the rooftops, but the rounds didn't penetrate. I have pictures of one that landed next to buildings, and you can see how the blast pattern had peppered the building with small fragments; but unless you were in the radius of the blast or out in the open, chances are you're going to be fine. I told my superiors, "We're okay where we're at. If we put sandbags on the windows in the event of an attack and take cover and stay low until it's over, we'll be fine." And we were. Nobody got hurt or injured as a result of any enemy activity while we were there at our surgical company. It's a good thing.

I came back to my medical-surgical unit in San Diego, and that's where I am now. A Marine we treated in Iraq stopped by the ward here one day. One of his responsibilities while out there was to check the runway for debris prior to the beginning of flight operations. They would look for trash that could get sucked up into the jet engine or damage the rotor blades of a helicopter. While he was doing this, unknowingly he picked up a high intensity flare that is used to throw a heat-seeking missile off its intended aerial target. They use these flares with chaff, which are like pieces of aluminum foil, to try and throw off the warhead. He picked it up, and it exploded in his hands causing full thickness burns across both palm areas and all of his fingers. He was immediately medevaced to Wilford Hall Army Medical Center in Texas for treatment of those burns and ended up staying there for two or three months. He said he has no feeling in his hands, but he can use his fingers. He came up to say, "Hi," which is very cool. You see guys like this from time to time.

I ran into a corpsman that had been in Iraq. An IED blew up next to his Humvee on one of the highways. When he came in he said, "Hey, I'm okay, doc — don't need anything. I can't hear anything out of my left ear, but I'm all right." Now he's got more continuing problems other than just a perforated ear drum.

Between my enlisted time and my officer time I have 20 years in service. I would be up to staying in for 30 years, but it depends on what the Navy decides to do with me. I have a package in to attend an "out-service" graduate program this year. It's a master's program in nursing administration. The selection process is very difficult with the Nurse Corps only picking up one or two to attend school. If I get selected, that would be great. If not, I may extend for a year and see what the Navy and the Nurse Corps can offer me as far as my next assignment. If I'm not picked up in January, it only gives me five or six months to negotiate for new orders, which within that window most of the good assignments are taken already. Hopefully they'll let me stay for another year. I like where I'm at. I like the flexibility and challenge of it. I'm an adrenaline junky, so I need that from time to time. To put me in an office someplace punching on a computer without human interaction would kill me. Most importantly, leadership is a privilege, and I'll take it any day of the week over any other job that you or the Navy can offer me.

MARGARET ARMSTRONG

Captain Margaret (Peg) Armstrong (Ret.) served in the United States Navy Nurse Corps for 38 years. She has cared for hundreds of patients. Her ability to synthesize information into sound statements of concise thought, prioritize tasks and make decisions has impacted the professional lives of hundreds of military nurses.

Peg learned from such masters of nursing as Lucy Germaine, director of nursing service at Harper Hospital, associate director of that hospital, director of the associated school of nursing, and editor and chief of the American Journal of Nursing. Peg cared for such notables as Miss Dubose, an original member of the United States Navy's Sacred Twenty, the original twenty members of the Navy Nurse Corps, and for Admiral Chester Nimitz.

Peg has been a member of the nursing faculty at several colleges or departments of nursing. These include University of Iowa, University of Washington, University of Utah and Old Dominion University. She advanced from ensign to captain. She has served as a Navy reserve unit training officer, commanding officer, assistant director of nursing service at a major naval medical facility and deputy director of the United States Navy Nurse Corps under three different directors of the United States Navy Nurse Corps. All of this experience and more clearly prepared Margaret Armstrong for the role she played during Operation Desert Storm. The following is only part of her story.

When I went to the University of Utah in 1981, I was teaching in the graduate program. I went to the Salt Lake City Navy reserve center where they had medical units. The units were in the process of growing. There was a lack of willingness on the part of the reserve center and the readiness command to consider nurses as executive (XO) and commanding officers (CO) of units. I happened to know that Admiral Francis Shea, director of the Navy Nurse Corps, had just started making this happen on active duty side. The active duty Navy ranks had changed to make it possible for nurses to hold these positions. I talked to the reserve center commanding officer and the readiness command; they said that it wasn't allowed. They said that it couldn't happen in the reserve until it happened on active duty. I told them, "Well, it is happening on active duty, sir."

After I went to my first selection board, I continued to inquire every other year all the way through the time I lived in Utah, for the lieutenant-lieutenant commander board for Navy Nurse Corps. Then I started going to the lieutenant-lieutenant commander selection boards for active duty, because they had to have one spot for reservists on their active duty boards. It meant that every other year I was going for the active boards and every other year I was going to the reserve board. When I started going to the active duty board, I met active duty nurses. I met nurses who had been in Vietnam and started hearing some of their stories. I also got to know wonderful people on active duty with the Nurse Corps and built friendships. Every year I had at least one selection board to go to, in addition to the regular two week active duty (AT).

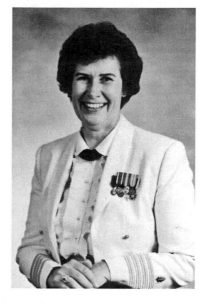

At the end of my time in Rochester, pay billets started going away. In looking for two-week active duty (AT) opportunities, I ended up going to the National Defense University for an AT. It was a great experience getting to know people in the "line" Navy. It was a two-week version of the one year National Defense

Margaret Armstrong graduated from Wayne State University in 1961 with a bachelor's degree in nursing. That same summer she entered the active duty United States Navy Nurse Corps as an ensign. After an amazing 38-year career in the Corps, she retired as a captain in May 1999.

University course that they sent active duty officers to. There were probably 500 going at a time. There were two women there the first time I went. The next year I was asked to come back for three weeks as a group leader. That was another great experience. Most were captains in the group for which I was a group leader. The Defense University was sort of a stepping stone in the reserve for line people.

Out of those experiences, I had collegial relationships with many active duty people. When I was told in Salt Lake City that nurses could not be in command of a unit and that I had no documentation that it was happening in the active duty or line community, it was very easy for me to make a couple of phone calls to the Bureau of Personnel (BUPERS) and to the Navy Nurse Corps to get a letter of support verifying that this was indeed happening on active duty. BUPERS agreed with me that they should send this documentation to all the readiness commands in the reserve. This made it possible for Navy Nurse Corps officers in the reserve to apply and be considered for CO and XO billets. Consequently, I became the CO of one of the reserve units. There were some problems with that on the part of a few of the men in the unit, partly because of their culture, partly because of their background and information. They could not see themselves reporting to a woman. One tried as hard as he could but couldn't adjust and very respectfully asked to transfer to the other unit.

We did several things to augment the learning and military activities of the unit, with the hope of attracting and keeping good people in the unit. At that time we were loaning corpsmen to the Seabees to go into the field with them. So we asked the Seabees to agree that in return they would go out with us on a weekend once or twice a year to teach our medical personnel how to safely handle and shoot firearms. With the beginning of fleet hospital, one had to know how to handle weapons safely and how to disarm them. It would also be useful not to panic, getting used to being around the sound of gunfire and not letting that hurt your efficiency and functioning. Little did I know at the time, that later nurses would carry firearms themselves when they were deployed. My ulterior motive was to increase the respect on the part of some of the men for the women in the medical unit. I knew, from people in the line, that women normally shoot better in the beginning than men do, because of their fine hand-eye coordination. For inexperienced people learning to shoot for the first time, normally the women do better. That would surprise some people, and that was my own ulterior motive.

The medical units grew, and the unit that I happened to be assigned to was the medical unit assigned to a hospital. Then it became a Pearl Harbor, Hawaii, unit which made it very easy to recruit people to join the reserve to be able to go to Hawaii for their reserve activity. After that it became a fleet hospital unit. Therefore, we did some survival training. And then it switched over to be a hospital ship Mercy unit. The unit had a variety of experiences, which was great fun.

It was later deemed illegal to have reserve units as support units for a hospital ship. Reservists could not legally be required to mobilize as quickly as a hospital ship was going to mobilize. Reservists had to be given a certain number of days to prepare to mobilize, and the hospital ships were required to be ready to deploy before that number of days. I think it was ten days, but I can't remember the exact number. That didn't make sense in the future because hospital ships never have left with their full complement of staff. They have always left with part of the complement later to be augmented. That turned out to be the way it happened in Desert Storm.

When I moved to Utah, I got a surprise phone call from one of my active duty colleagues. I was going to the Chautauqua Nursing Conference every year, and the current deputy director of the Navy Nurse Corps, Madeline Ancelard, was also going to Chautauqua. I had just moved to Utah. My stuff wasn't even unpacked yet. She asked if I would go to Washington on active duty to be in the office of assistant secretary of defense, Reserve Affairs. I said, "There is no way I can do that, ethically. The University of Utah just paid for me to move to Utah. I just signed a contract to teach here. I cannot now, after being here for one week, tell them I am going back on active duty." She said, "Peg, this opportunity is very rare to come along." The other thing I had just found out, as I was moving into my house in Utah, is that I was selected for captain. She said, "We never call back captains to active duty. This is never going to happen again." I said, "I can't help it. I can't be unethical." She said, "Who would you recommend?" I said, "I would recommend Captain Pauline Kominich. She would be perfect for that job." Madeline did call her and Pauline did go back on active duty. Pauline then went to the University of Arizona.

I went on my merry way with the medical unit I have described. I continued to go to selection boards. While I was in Utah, the Navy Nurse Corps decided that they would have a one week AT in the Bureau of Medicine (BUMED) for commanders and captains in the reserve to give them an overview. In the past, when Admiral Maxine Condor was director of the Navy Nurse Corps, she knew there were reservists. When I visited Admiral Condor one time she said, "I know we have reservists and I know they are very talented. I would certainly like to use them, but I'm not sure how."

The next director of the Navy Nurse Corps was Admiral Francis Shea. Admiral Shea left active duty, was a drilling reservist in Chicago for a few years, and went back to active duty. This was in the day of few pay billets. She knew the problems the reservists had finding meaningful experiences. She was very supportive. She cracked the door open. She started having a reservist that lived locally coming in and doing projects at BUMED in the Nurse Corps office. When she turned over to Admiral Mary Nielubowicz as director of Navy Nurse Corps, she pushed for Admiral Nielubowicz to continue that project.

When Admiral Nielubowicz was limited in the amount of funding she had to do the things she wanted to do for the active duty Nurse Corps, she did things where she could. One of the things she did was push the door wide open and start bringing reservists in and really started to utilize them. It was her idea to bring senior Nurse Corps officers in for a week to get an overview. We had briefs to get an overview of what was going on in the Navy and the Nurse Corps. This was because these were senior people in the reserve. Anyone that wanted to could stay on for a second week and work in the Nurse Corps office to get their full two-week AT, which is what I did. There were four of us that did that. We had to fill out a little card with our background and our graduate course work. Afterward, during a break, Captain Anita Sheehan, the deputy director of the Navy Nurse Corps came in and said, "Captain Armstrong, you come with me. I need you!" I had written postgraduate work in rehab. She said, "The theme of the federal Nurses' Day program at meetings of the Society of the Federal Health Agencies (AMSUS) is going to be rehab, and I want you to be the master of ceremonies for the program that day. We're having a planning committee meeting with the Air Force and the Army this afternoon. You are coming with me." All of that happened just because I had taken those courses. I said, "OK, yes, ma'am." The three last names of the directors of the military Nurse Corps were Admiral Nielubowicz, Brigadier General Slewitzke, and Brigidier General Shimmenti. They were impressed because I pronounced their names correctly all day long.

The second week the four of us worked in the Nurse Corps office. Captain Sheehan knew nothing about computers. She had a few letters that came in with questions. She said, "Can anyone use a computer?" I raised my hand and wrote the answers to letters. That was the first time that they had had an experience with a reservist doing specific things that were helpful to them in the Navy Nurse Corps office.

In 1983, the Navy Nurse Corps had their first program at AMSUS. I gave a presentation about writing fitness reports. That was Admiral Nielubowicz's first AMSUS. She really reached out to the reserve officers, and it was the beginning of a long process. It wasn't more than five years later when there were 500 Navy Nurses going to AMSUS on orders. It was a major educational opportunity.

A couple of years later at AMSUS something happened that was the result of Admiral Nielubowicz's interest in the reserve. Because of becoming acquainted with reserve officers at that conference at BUMED and as a result of her first and second year at AMSUS, she made a decision that she needed to go New Orleans in person to talk to the flag officers directing the reserve medical programs. She took Captain Sheehan with her as the deputy director of the Navy Nurse Corps to get acquainted and express their interest in having more participation of the reserve Nurse Corps officers with the active duty Nurse Corps. That never happened before and has never happened since.

For years there had been a reserve flag officer council. It was made up of flag officers in the Medical Corps (MC) and the Dental Corps (DC) reserve with no representative from the Medical Service Corps (MSC) or Nurse Corps (NC). They met three times a year on paid orders for weekends, and they developed policies for the medical department reserve with only two out of the four corps represented at the meetings (MC and DC). It is little wonder that the Nurse Corps and the MSC were not getting needed legislation initiated to meet their needs as naval officers. Admiral Nielubowicz campaigned to have at least one senior member of the Nurse Corps and Medical Service Corps on the council.

The following year at AMSUS, the admiral from New Orleans who was in charge of the medical reserve was giving a talk. Admiral Nielubowicz and I were sitting in the front row. I will never forget that day. He said, "Admiral Nielubowicz, I want to extend to you the invitation to choose someone from the reserve Nurse Corps to be a representative on the flag council." The meeting broke for lunch. She said, "Peg, I will meet you in the dining room" (where the Navy medical reserve luncheon was being held). She said, "I'm going to go right in and get a table and I want you to go around the room and gather up every reserve Nurse Corps officer captain and bring them to that table. We are going to pick a person now so that after lunch I will go back and tell him who our representative is. We have to strike while the iron is hot, because everyone in this room heard what he said. If we wait, he'll say, 'That's not what I meant.'" There were about 12 Nurse Corps reserve captains there. The waitress came around getting our orders. As I had my head turned ordering my iced tea, I could hear Admiral Nielubowicz saying to the group, "I want your input right now. I want you to be thinking and by the end of the time we finish eating, I want you to tell me who in your community around the country should be the Nurse Corps representative on the reserve flag council." I turned my head back from ordering my iced tea to pay attention to the discussion that was about to take place. Admiral Nielubowicz said, "Well then, that's settled. Captain Armstrong you will be the representative for the reserve flag council." I said, "Admiral, aren't we going to discuss that?" She said, "We just did." That's how it happened. Then we proceeded to have our lunch. I was sitting there thinking, "What just happened? What does this mean?" We reconvened at the Navy reserve medical meeting and Admiral Nielubowicz informed Admiral Summit that the representative to the flag council would be Captain Armstrong and she was to have orders to the next flag council meeting. I later found out that everyone at the table pointed to me while I was ordering my iced tea.

About that same time my tour as CO of the medical unit in Salt Lake was coming to an end. Admiral Nielubowicz had Captain Sheehan call me about a reserve unit based at the Pentagon. It was a CNO unit. They had a billet available. Captain Sheehan said, "If you are willing to travel to D.C. to drill, I would like you to get a billet in that unit but drill at BUMED in the Navy Nurse Corps office." That's what I did. I consolidated my drills and did all my drills for each quarter at one time in the Nurse Corps office. I drilled six days at a time. One of those quarters I also did my AT attached to my six days. I started getting very well acquainted with the people at BUMED, the politics, the contacts and so on.

When I started there, the retention rate in the Navy Nurse Corps reserve community was about 60 percent. In other words, about 40 percent left every year. There was a decrease in pay billets to the point that there were so few pay billets in the country that people were either getting out of the reserve or they were transferring to the Army or Air Force where they could get pay billets. The reserve community in the Navy Nurse Corps was down to about 887. A very small percentage actually had pay billets. Many people were transferring to VTUs (voluntary training units). The number of billets that were actually filled was 56 percent. Consequently, the deputy surgeon general was pressuring Admiral Nielubowicz to start accepting associate degree nurses into the reserve as commissioned Nurse Corps officers. He wanted to give them an accession incentive with educational support to get their degrees if they did not have a pay billet where they lived. The problem was you couldn't have associate degree nurses as commissioned officers on active duty. That was not a problem to those people because they would only mobilize and bring them on active duty in case of war and then it would be acceptable. Admiral Nielubowicz did not want to do that. None of it made sense, but she was getting a lot of pressure. Admiral Nielubowicz said, "Peg, I want your first project to be to write a paper, not only rebutting that proposal, but also tell me what is needed to bring the manning level up and increase retention."

They sent another captain to work with me. We spent two weeks interviewing people around Washington. The morning I arrived, Captain Sheehan said, "You're coming with me! I have an appointment lined up with the deputy surgeon general. Then you are going to see the director of Navy reserve (who was actually in the Pentagon). I'm driving you over but I'm not going in with you because we don't get along and I would rip his face off if I had to look at him." I thought, "Oh my! He must not be a very nice person." I'm dumped into the deputy surgeon general's office by myself. The deputy surgeon general was from New Jersey. He was like a New Jersey street fighter, really, with a lot of gumption. He was peppering me with questions: Why should we do this? Why should we do that? Why can't we do it this way? And this is an easy fix to bring in associate degree nurses. I went to see the director of the Navy reserve, who kind of gave me the same approach. As I am leaving his office, Admiral Neil Smith, who was the deputy director of Navy reserve at the time, came out of his office, into the hallway behind me, and said, "You're Captain Armstrong and you've come here to work on this project for Admiral Nielubowicz, correct?" I said, "Yes." He said, "You go captain. You show them that is not the thing to do." I said, "That's interesting. OK. Yes sir." I found out later that his wife was a retired Navy nurse. He later became the director of the Navy reserve and was the main force in the Pentagon behind our getting a flag billet for Nurse Corps officers later on.

We interviewed over 100 people either by phone or in person. We gathered data from the individuals and organizations. The next time I went back to Washington I used the data to write a point paper suggesting the legislation we needed. We needed scholarship money, an older age for accession, and a loan repayment program. The strategy was that we didn't need to lower our standards. We needed to increase our standards to attract qualified people. Of course, we also needed the pay billets back. They were beginning to come back because of the work of an MSC officer in the reserve office at BUMED who wrote point papers to get the pay billets back. He was taking care of that piece at that time. My point paper with graphs was written. Now Admiral Nielubow-icz had what she needed to take around as a rebuttal.

One morning back in Utah, I got a call again from Captain Sheehan. She said, "Well, good morning, Captain Armstrong. I have been waiting three hours to call you." Captain Sheehan arrived at work at about four in the morning. Of course, being two hours later than Washington, she waited a long time. As it was, she probably called at six-thirty or seven my time in Utah. She said, "Well, Captain Armstrong," and she always called me Peg. We were good friends by that time. She said, "The postman is ringing for the second time, believe it or not. I'm calling you once more to ask if you would be willing to come back on active duty fulltime." She said, "Admiral Nielubowicz wants you here all the time, not just part time. She has taken a billet from Jacksonville, has moved it to Bethesda, and it is to be used for a new billet at BUMED. She wants to have a second deputy director of the Nurse Corps: one for active duty and one for reserve. She wants you to come and get the legislation passed that is needed, increase the retention and get these billets filled." (The billet numbers then were up to about 2,800, but we still had only 1,100 people in the reserve Nurse Corps.) She said, "Can you consider it this time?" I said, "Yes, I believe I can." I had been at the University full time from 1981–1986.

The wheels were put in motion. I got a call that I remember very distinctly from Captain Dottie Leonard, who was in charge of the accession board at BUMED. I had been on her board when she was selected for captain. Dottie Leonard called me and said, "Peg, your paperwork is completed. You've been accepted. You're reporting date for BUMED is such and such. You'll be getting your orders in the mail." She said, "I only have one last thing to tell you," and she started to laugh. Then she started the sentence again and started to laugh again. She couldn't complete the sentence. This went on several times. I said, "Dottie, for goodness sake, what are you trying to tell me?" She said, "I am trying to tell you that normally when we bring people back on active duty, if it has been more than five years after that they have been off of active duty, they have to go back to Newport and go through officer indoctrination." She said, "None of us could fathom you doing that." She said, "You have been a captain now for seven years, and we can't see you as a captain back at Newport." The image struck her so funny. She said, "You're exempt." I said, "I never knew it was a requirement, so I am glad to hear that I am exempt."

The dean of the college of nursing at the University of Utah offered me a leave of absence. I said, "That wouldn't be fair." At that point, I thought I was going back on active duty for two years. "I wouldn't mind you keeping the position open for one year, but two years wouldn't be fair for the school." Off I went to Washington and found an apartment.

Normally in the Washington environment in the government, it takes a full year to figure out who the people are that you are working with and who the contacts are that you can trust, what the language is all about, etc. It didn't take me more than three or four months because I had 18 months already working in that environment part time. It ended up being anywhere from the equivalent of eight to twelve weeks per year during that period of time. I had a head start, you might say. They asked me what I needed in that job. I said I needed an 800 phone number so I could communicate with the reserve community and a desk. I should have been a little more grandiose because when I got there that is literally all I had. The desk was a wooden desk with one wobbly leg. It only had one drawer. My officemate found it in the hallway. I had the 800 number, but that was it. That was the crucial thing to ask for. That 800 number is still there, even though a few people have tried to get rid of it.

Here is where my public speaking experience and my dealing with cantankerous people who didn't want you to accomplish your goals came in handy. I was never a political person but I learned very quickly. I eventually had my own office and quickly had reserve Nurse Corps officers coming for their ATs, one, two, three at a time; 200 to 300 a year. After I was there for about three months, the legislation that had been worked on between my counterparts in the Army and Air Force actually came through as legislation as one big package. I was so excited. I could hardly stay in my skin. Captain Sheehan said, "I really don't understand why you're so excited." She couldn't appreciate what all those things meant: the loan repayment program, the stipend program, the increase in the age for accession, and so on. I said, "You realize, Captain, this affects all of the people on active duty as well as those who are United States Navy reserve." Oh, wait a minute! That took on a whole different complexion.

Captain Sheehan left in December and Captain Swetonik had come into the office. Admiral Nielubowicz had turned over to Admiral Hall, who had not had much experience with the Nurse Corps reserve. I reported onboard about three weeks before Admiral Hall did. Admiral Nielubowiez told Admiral Hall, "The reserve is an important part of your responsibility as director of Navy Nurse Corps. You have this valuable community and they are ready to serve as needed."

Admiral Hall started asking for people from the reserve community to come on active duty to contribute things that she needed to accomplish. For example, there had never been a complete analysis of the billet structure in the active duty Navy Nurse Corps. In other words, there had never been an analysis of which billets were occurring with which NOBCs or specialty codes, at what rank, what clinical specialties and if that was the mix that they needed. She said, "I have manpower experts but not anyone who can analyze the whole community. Do you know of anybody in the reserve?" I said, "We have a reservist who's a captain who has spent the last five years doing the national manpower analysis studies for the Association of Colleges of Nursing, and she lives here in Washington D.C. I happen to know that she is getting bored with her job." She said, "Let's bring her on active duty!"

Susan Jackson came on active duty. In one year, she did the first complete billet analysis in the Navy Nurse Corps. That gave the Nurse Corps the basis upon which to do total billet realignment to determine what they needed for Marine support units, fleet hospitals, for everything that they now knew they had and how they needed to change. It is a complicated mix, not just numbers and ranks. She was one of the many people that we brought back on active duty. We had to bring her back while BUPERS would allow it to happen at the senior ranks. We brought a reservist back on active duty full time to be a reserve liaison officer with each of the big four naval hospitals to increase the collegiality and input and participation of reserve Nurse Corps officers in those facilities for drilling, not just for their AT. That came in very handy when Desert Storm came along because those people were in place to coordinate bringing reservists onboard. They knew who their assets were in reserve units coming into the hospitals.

There were people that were coming back onto active duty in senior positions that had a big influence, not just in Washington, but also in different places around the country. We started putting reserve officers on readiness command (REDCOM) staffs as reservists, not on active duty. At the same time, there was a person that was my counterpart in the Air Force director of the Nurse Corps office, Irene Trowell-Harris. She was a colonel in the Air Force National Guard. We started meeting on a regular basis. Then the director of the Army Nurse Corps office got someone. Reserve Affairs in the Pentagon had someone from the Army who was in Reserve Affairs in manpower to look at all services. We began to meet as a group, sometimes weekly, sometimes monthly. Anything you wanted to get through Congress had to be for all the services, not just one. We all had to be in unison so our proposals would be supported on all fronts.

By the time I left Washington five years later, the reserve group numbered 20 who had fulltime, active duty billets in the three services. Then it included the flag officers because the Army reserve got a flag officer as did the Air Force reserve. Through working with Admiral Neil Smith, who was now the director of Navy reserve, we were able to get the flag billets through with the help of Senator Znouye. In the meanwhile, I was still on the flag council along with an MSC reservist. When I went back on active duty, I stayed on the flag council. This helped a great deal in getting support and for them to at least be aware of what we were doing. The MSC representative, who was an optometrist with whom I had a very good working relationship, said to me, "You are going to be able to do a lot more on active duty for the Nurse Corps getting a flag billet than we are. We don't have a full-time reservist on active duty in Washington." I said, "We are not just campaigning for the Nurse Corps. We will not accept a billet for the Navy Nurse Corps unless we get it for the Medical Service Corps. We are going as a package." That created unity between MSC and the Navy Nurse Corps reserve officers.

We ended up creating a three-pronged pressure front, and we coordinated it at the same time to get those two flag billets established. Admiral Neil Smith from his position in the Pentagon, his legislative affairs person, as well as the legislative affairs person in the secretary of the Navy's office, and Senator Znouye proposed the billets be established. Senator Znouye ended up telling the surgeon general that if he did not instruct the reserve flag council to give up two of its own billets, one for Navy Medical Service Corps (MSC) and one for the Navy Nurse Corps, he would personally do a review of the flag officer billet structure in the medical reserve. That meant they took the risk of losing more than one for each corps. They finally condescended to give one billet for Navy Nurse Corps and one for the MSC.

Things were going along pretty well. Retention was starting to come up. Numbers were coming up. REDCOMS were asking me to visit. I was traveling one to three weekends a month, which was a pleasure. People were coming in the office and then taking the word back about what was going on. People were at least getting informed, and through AMSUS, getting acquainted with each other. The REDCOM staff nurses were meeting and becoming acquainted. There was a council of REDCOM staff nurses. Then we met at AMSUS and there would be a full day of meetings before AMSUS even started with all the REDCOM staff nurses. The four liaison officers from the four major hospitals would come; a lot of key people, including all the people that were on active duty in special billets from the reserve. We would talk about reserve issues and what we needed to do next, what we needed to accomplish. It was almost like a reserve Nurse Corps executive conference every year, which helped a lot.

In January of 1990, the surgeon general called Admiral Hall and said he had to see both of us in his office. He said, "I have been given the order by the chief of naval operations (CNO) to remove $40 million from my budget." There were a lot of budget cuts that year. That was the beginning of downsizing. He said, "I have to decrease my overall budget $40 million without affecting service to our beneficiaries. The only place that I can do that without affecting the care in the hospitals, deployments and overseas billets is in the reserve. So I have eliminated the budget, starting 1 October this year for the next fiscal year, for the hospital backfill half of the medical reserve." That would eliminate all billets that were not fleet hospital or Marine or air support.

Air had no regular pay billets so they didn't have any real billets. They always got their people from other programs. He said, "I cannot do it to the Marine support units. I cannot do it to the fleet hospital units. If I eliminate billets in the reserve fleet hospital program, then I am going to be given this question: If you don't need the reserve fleet hospitals then how many active duty fleet hospitals do you need? As long as I say I need this many reserve (fleet hospitals), obviously I need this many active duty. You have to understand that the mobilization billets are the funding basis for active duty billets. Every active duty officer in the staff corps has a mobilization billet. That's what provides the funds for that billet. If you take away an active duty fleet hospital, that means you take away the number of billets to staff a 500 or 1,000 bed hospital. That means those active duty billets disappear."

He said, "Captain Armstrong, I did this last week. I am waking up at night in a cold sweat. What's going to happen in my hospitals in case of war and there are no reservists to come to backfill the people who are being deployed? You've got to do something." He wasn't cutting our throat. It was just that he had no other place to cut money from. He had no wiggle room. What was he going to do, cut $40 million out of the active duty budget? That would certainly affect service to beneficiaries. That was his direct order. He didn't call in the admiral of medical reserve. I said, "Admiral, why are you saying this to me?" He said, "Because you are the only medical reservist with experience here fulltime at BUMED." He said, "Will you do what you can? We have to get $40 million back in the budget. But when you go to people for support to find $40 million someplace, they are going to say, 'Why should I do it when your sponsor made the cut himself. Surgeon general is the one who took it out.'" I don't know why I said this, but I said, "Admiral, I am going to take care of this." I walked out of his office saying to myself, "Who in the hell did you think you were saying that you were going to do your best to take care of this?" He said, "You have to realize, Captain Armstrong, I cannot be involved in the process because I was the one that removed the item from the budget. In other words, you cannot invoke my name." I said, "I will not use your name. I will not involve you in the process. I will not even tell you what I am doing, but I promise I will not do anything illegal." He said, "I can't ask for anything more than that."

I was used to working 12 to 14 hours a day. I had not finished my dissertation because of taking care of my mother. On the personal side, when I first went to Washington, I went to George Mason University in their doctoral program in nursing administration and was taking two courses at a time. I don't know how I was doing it. It was always hard with two or three incompletes trying to finish all my work. When this happened with the budget problem, I just said this is just not going to work. I can't do this assignment and the regular things that were time-consuming, traveling one to three weekends a month and take care of the budget problem as well.

I had two dear friends, one civilian and the other a Navy colleague. We were at the Pentagon City Mall. I sat down and said, "I have to quit school. I

cannot finish the doctoral program and do all that I have to do for the Navy."
They both jumped up and down saying, "Hooray, hooray!" I was driving
myself crazy trying to do that.

There was a set of congressional budget hearings coming up for the following fiscal year in about eight weeks. There was no time to go through
official channels to get data to document the need for the $40 million. My first
thought was that we had to document what the medical reservists and the
medical backfill units were already doing in peacetime was worth. If they are
not worth $40 million in peacetime, they are not worth keeping in case of war.
But I didn't have time to do a detailed study. I called the admiral in charge of
the Navy reserve in New Orleans, and I called Admiral Smith, director of
reserve for the whole Navy. I said, "I need permission to use your name to say
we don't have time to get this done through official channels, but this is the
data I need." They both gave me permission. I went to the secretary of the
Navy office and couldn't find anybody to help support me, because they all
said, "Look, the sponsor took the money out. It was his decision." I found one
captain in the secretary of the Navy office who would help me. I found one
colonel who was an Army Nurse Corps officer who was a recalled reservist in
the office of the assistant secretary of defense for Reserve Affairs who understood the politics of the issues, Sheila Bowman. She had been in our tri-service
group and knew me. She had been working in Pentagon policy for several
years. It was her boss that the Navy medicine budget people had to report to
regarding the overall reserve budget.

We went to work. We called every hospital and facility where medical
reservists drilled and performed AT, to the reserve offices where people
reported and the reserve liaison offices. We asked for the man hours of corpsmen, dental techs, physicians, nurses, and MSC officers for the past two quarters. There is not going to be any backfill starting October 1st if we don't prove
that our contributed man hours are worth at least $40 million. We don't have
time to do it the normal way of business. Everyone cooperated.

Interestingly enough, when the admiral in charge of the reserve office at
BUMED found out what was going on, he made an appointment with the
director of the Nurse Corps, Admiral Hall. He did this in order to beg her that
those statistics not be reported by corps, but be all lumped together in the
total. She had already seen the rough figures and she knew why he was asking.
He knew what those statistics showed, that the Nurse Corps officers in the
reserve were spending far more time in the hospitals and the clinics than the
physicians. He didn't want the figure to stand out for the physicians. She did
not agree to do that.

I took all the preliminary statistics to the people who supported us. The
captain in the secretary of the Navy's office said they needed to personally
visit Bethesda. "We need to just look at one of the large facilities to see if this

is valid data. I'm not saying you doctored the data. The data showed that the hospital units were contributing more than $40 million a year in care hours. We need to say that we made one site visit and that this is valid accurate data." We arranged a meeting for them. Yes, indeed it was true. In the meanwhile, when one of the comptrollers at BUMED, who reported to the assistant secretary of defense for Reserve Affairs, would be required to go over and answer questions about budget, he would never bring anything written. He would only bring verbal reports, but he was required to put in monthly budgetary and activity reports every month to Reserve Affairs. I routinely got copies of those reports. Colonel Bowman said, "If I could know what is written down, because all the facts were there documenting the need for these units, I could brief my boss so he would know what questions to ask of Captain so-and-so." We got into a routine, almost every two weeks of meetings in the Pentagon parking lot on my way into work to give her the copy of the official reports he had to hand in at BUMED. He was beginning to be put on the spot with pointed questions, so he had to give them the information and validate what they already knew. These were the different things going on, nothing illegal. Those are reports they should have been getting anyway, but he never took them over.

The last week in July before going on leave to Utah, I got the phone call from the secretary of the Navy office that $40 million was being taken from the line budget and being put back into Navy medicine for the backfill positions of the medical reserve. Three days later on August 1, Sadam Hussein invaded Kuwait. If that $40 mil hadn't gone back in the budgets after 1 October, there would have been no reservists to mobilize. That program would have been completely gone. I felt that all that work was well, well worth it. It took the cooperation of a lot people doing things outside the normal way of doing business. It was a wonderful feeling!

I was in Utah when I heard about Sadam Hussein invading Kuwait. That night I had a dream, and the next morning told my friends, "I had a dream that just didn't make sense." Because all it was, was a blurb on the news that Sadam Hussein has gone into Kuwait, nothing about the United States. They are mobilizing troops along the border and going to Kuwait. I had a dream that the United States was going to war in Kuwait. There were a lot of things going on in the world that we weren't getting involved in. The hospital ships were going, and it was like a nightmare.

The following week I went to the Chautauqua Nursing Conference on my way back to Washington. Admiral Hall was there. I was giving a full-day workshop on stress management, and during the morning break someone came in and said, "I have to make an announcement. All Air Force nurses attending the conference at Chautauqua are to pack up and leave and report to their commands tomorrow. They are to leave Vail today." I thought that was interesting. Something's going on in the Air Force. When I broke for lunch, somebody came and said that Admiral Hall wanted to see me immediately in the cafeteria. She said, "I just got a call that the Comfort and the Mercy are going out. We're going to leave tomorrow instead of the day after."

I was driving Admiral Hall from Vail back to Denver to get our plane. She said we would probably be mobilizing the reserve, etc., etc. She said, "How do you feel about this? Do you think we are ready to go?" I said, "Yes." By that time, our numbers had gone from about 1,100 to 2,750 people. We had a 93 percent retention rate. About 98 percent of the billets were filled. Obviously, there was no more pressure to lower our standards. I said, "How do I feel about this? Admiral Hall, my only fear about coming back on active duty is that something like this would happen and I would be stuck in an office." She said, "My dear, that is exactly what's happened."

When the first cadre for the Comfort and Mercy left we did a 75 percent backfill with mobilization of reservists. In other words, if a 100 people left Bethesda, 75 reservists went in. The rationale being that many of the collateral duties would not be happening in wartime, so we did not need a 100 percent replacement. You might if they started to receive casualties, but at that point they didn't.

For whatever psychological reason, the deputy director of the Navy Nurse Corps for the active duty side was really not interested in what was going on in Desert Storm. I think it might have had something to do with her Vietnam experience. It was, for some reason, something that she could not deal with. Very quickly she took care of the normal active duty Navy Nurse Corps business and I took care of the reserve, plus whatever was going on that was different because of the war. That was mainly the mobilization of the reserves and integration of the reserve Navy Nurse Corps officers going into the hospitals, determining how many numbers, working with the directors of nursing service (DNS) at the hospitals and what was happening with the reserve offices, how many were leaving, and how many reservists were needed.

New Orleans was quite slow in getting underway to meet the manpower of Desert Shield Desert Storm. What happened has not happened with Iraqi Freedom or any of the other deployments of reservists since. We decided at the reserve office at BUMED (not the Nurse Corps office), that we needed a cadre of people quickly to coordinate the mobilization of the reserve physicians, corpsmen and nurses. We brought a lieutenant commander back on active duty from the reserve from NHSETC. We called her to BUMED. I had a captain drilling in the office with me at the time for her consolidated drills, Judy Stagg. I said, "Judy, can you go home and come back in a week on active duty?" She said, "Excuse me?" She came back and didn't leave for five years. She eventually became the director of Reserve Affairs at BUMED, underneath the admiral, who was, of course, not there full time, as he was a drilling reservist.

We brought a couple of others on to active duty because they had already been drilling in my office. One was ordered to Reserve Affairs and the other stayed with me in the office. We brought in several other people. One gal from Rhode Island came because she was a REDCOM staff nurse. I knew her and knew she wanted to come back on active duty anyway. There ended up with about eight Nurse Corps reserve officers mobilized within a week. Those eight people literally coordinated the mobilization of everyone from the Reserve Medical Department for Desert Shield/Desert Storm. Another joined them to help with the manpower pieces.

When the mobilization was complete, 1,560 reserve nurses had been mobilized, three by name for specific reasons; one as department head for critical care for a fleet hospital, one for post–traumatic stress management for a fleet hospital ended up being on the SPRINT team at the barracks at Dhahran when it was hit by a SCUD missile, and one as assistant director of nursing service of one of the two fleet hospitals. All the rest were mobilized by computer by area and REDCOM. We left several REDCOM's untouched on purpose. One was REDCOM 10, in the panhandle of Florida and Louisiana. The others were the Minnesota REDCOM and the Great Lakes REDCOM. These were set aside because we knew there might be other needs later on. We did pull people out of the Texas group for specific needs, like with the Marines, because they had many male nurses that were very experienced with trauma. We also knew that the hospital ships might eventually need reserve augmentation. I used to get calls from the REDCOM staff nurse in New Orleans saying, "Captain, no one in my REDCOM has been mobilized." I said, "Just have some patience. Your time will come. Just have people ready. But we don't need them now."

We mobilized twice the number of Nurse Corps officers as we did Medical Corps officers. We mobilized four times the number of officers of any other reserve community in the Navy. Not one out of the 1,560 refused to go. There were a few that couldn't go because they were in the first trimester of pregnancy. We had people who had just left active duty the week before and were in the process of moving. We had people that just joined the Navy reserve a month or two before. We had people calling saying, "Captain, I have been mobilized; I have ten days to report, I have this situation, I need an extension of two more days." But it wasn't a matter of "I can't come." We had physicians who were refusing to go. Several Nurse Corps officers who were unit COs called saying, "I don't know what I can do with Dr. so-and-so or Captain so-and-so. He is refusing to go." We had Nurse Corps officers who were making six-figures, were mobilized, and went willingly. I had a set of parents call and say, "Our daughter is being mobilized to go to war and she can't go." I said, "Is she pregnant?" They said, "No." "Does she have a child that is critically ill?" "No." I went through the normal reasons. "Why can't she go?" "Because

we don't want her to go. She's our daughter, Captain. You have to understand."
I said, "Does she want to go?" "Oh, yes, she wants to go." I got some calls like
that that were very heartwarming.

It wasn't really until Desert Storm was almost over that the New Orleans
staff got in gear. They hadn't had to do that sort of thing for many decades.
When the mobilization piece was nearly finished, we did come to a point where
all of our available critical care nurses, operating room nurses, and nurse anesthetists were just about down to the bottom. The following week, we had identified members of the Individual Ready Reserve (IRR), inactive people that
were not drilling regularly. We were going to start dipping into the IRR to
mobilize when the ground war ended. Eventually, over Christmas, I did call
the REDCOM staff nurse in New Orleans and said, "You're going to send out
120 people along with another group because about 100 people are needed to
augment the staff of the two hospital ships."

In December and January the two reserve fleet hospitals were mobilized.
They went to Fort Dix for three weeks of training before they went to Desert
Storm. I spent six weeks at Fort Dix with them. One of the things I did was
to interview one-on-one every corpsman and Nurse Corps officer that had
been to Vietnam to make sure they were emotionally able to go. We sent a few
home. They were clearly in a panic mode and unable to function. A few were
fine. The other third I was really uncertain about, so we set up a good support
system for them so they would have two or three people keeping a close eye
on them, to give them the support they needed to make the adjustment, or if
they got into trouble, to let someone know.

There were several unique things that needed to be settled and things
you'd never think about. We had African American women going to the desert
for the duration. How were they to keep sanitized with their hair? Cornrows
were not yet permitted in uniform. They clearly needed to be able to have
their hair done in cornrows so that they could keep their heads clean, safe and
disease-free for up to six months. I went back to BUMED in between the two
fleet hospitals for a few days, and we made that request up to SECNAV, so I
could go back and get that settled before they left. I was at the terminal to see
every plane load of people leave. That was absolutely heart wrenching, but
heartwarming at the same time.

I can remember making rounds in the nurses' quarters the night before
they were to leave. There were some people that needed more buttons and
hangers. Before I went back to Washington, I called the reservist in the office
and said go around to the different dry cleaners and collect hangers. That was
my pretense for visiting them, to hand out hangers and buttons. They found
out that they weren't going to have a place to get those things. Obviously they
are going to lose a few buttons, and they didn't know for how long they were
going to be there.

One of the girls broke her leg one night dancing at the Officers' Club. She was heartbroken that they weren't going to let her go. They found out at the last minute that it was a stress fracture that would actually heal faster being on her feet with the walking cast that she had. So, she got to go. There was a lot of anxiety among both fleet hospital groups because there were older people that had been accessed because of the increase in accession age (the age at which nurses could join the military), who were very anxious about going to war. I convinced them of the reality that they were going to be able to function better than the younger nurses because all the equipment was old-fashioned, simple equipment; for example, old Gomco suction machines because they were easier to repair and easier to operate. The young nurses had never worked with some of that equipment. That turned out to be true. The other interesting dynamic regarding age was that after every class session broke up, you would see all the younger Nurse Corps officers and corpsmen gathering around the older women. It was as if each group had their mothers with them. These were women in their 40s and 50s. They became their emotional pillar. They would gather around them and just sit, wanting to be next to somebody older.

The night before the first fleet hospital left, I got a phone call because a group of 15 active duty nurses were being sent out to augment the reserve fleet hospitals. They were being sent out on the same planes. They arrived and I spent half the night with them, getting them up to speed with what was going on. That meant a lot to them.

About three-quarters of the way through the first group, I thought, "This is all getting much too serious." So I had a class with the Nurse Corps officers. I told them, "You haven't had orientation as to other things you need to be aware of." I knew from friends like Captain Loughney and Captain Carroll on the hospital ships about shopping and so forth. I told them that if they got a chance for liberty, where they could go shopping for gold, jewelry, rugs, etc. If you play golf, you can have a friend send you a two-foot square of artificial turf. You can go out and practice your golf swing in the desert. "Captain, how are we going to do that?" "You put your little piece of turf, or indoor/outdoor carpeting on the sand, hit the ball, pick up the turf and go and put it under the ball." It was an hour of that. Some of them thought I was absolutely out of my mind. We talked about keeping the control you could keep. You feel that all the control has been taken away from you, but you still have control over some things. When you get on the plane, you can decide whether you are going to sleep or stay awake. Focus on the things you do have control of. People are still reminding me of how bizarre they thought that was at the time, but how helpful the information was later.

People went to church services. The Catholics had a mass set up especially for them by the Catholic chaplains on base. Many non–Catholics went to pray together and be together for that hour of church.

When the nurses had their weekend off before leaving Fort Dix, I took the DNS and/or the ADNS and spent the weekend with them and get them away. In both situations, they felt a lot of responsibility. The one fleet hospital DNS did go home because she's from New Jersey and we were at Fort Dix. I went away with them for the weekend to Atlantic City. We had two full days to talk about leadership, responsibility, taking care of themselves, their mental health, etc. My biggest worry throughout the whole thing was that they would come back safely. That is basically all I cared about. I felt they'd function fine.

As the war was grinding to a halt, I got a call saying I had orders cut to relieve the director of nursing services for the active duty fleet hospital. Out of courtesy, I did suggest that the person in contingency planning notify Admiral Hall. She not only said, "No," but "Hell no!" They consequently changed their mind about relieving anybody in that fleet hospital because the ground war was about to start in a few days so that it did not happen. I had my sea bag ready. We all had our dog tags and immunizations; everybody on active duty, no matter who you were, was ready. As soon as Desert Storm happened, everybody had immunizations, lenses made for goggles; everything was done.

As soon as the ground war ended, I got a call from the surgeon general's office, which had gotten a call from the CO of the Comfort. They had some concerns that they had not done a history of the ship's mission and this was the first operational mission of the hospital ship. The Mercy had gone to the Philippines on a humanitarian mission, but this was the first wartime operational mission. The surgeon general had known, just because we used to talk, that I had taken historical research courses at George Mason University. It had come in handy for one reason, but it also came in handy for many administration pieces in my job. There was no more funding for sending people over there. The war was over. But the surgeon general, the same surgeon general for whom I saved $40 million, wanted to send me over there to sail back with the Comfort. I flew to Malaga, Spain, met the ship and spent a little more than three weeks on the ship on the way back to Baltimore, interviewing the part of the staff that had stayed onboard. I had three days to get ready once the decision was made. I took tapes and batteries and asked everyone standardized questions. I interviewed Nurse Corps officers, physicians, MSC officers, the CO and XO of the ship, reservists and MSTS personnel (what used to be called the Merchant Marine), down to the plumber.

After the ship got back, I went to the Comfort in Baltimore. They gave me their original photographs and videotapes. I took examples of all the different types of message traffic. That's all catalogued on acid-free paper and acid-free staples and the materials are now at the historical research floor of the Navy library at the Naval Yard in Washington D.C. That was a wonderful experience. Six months later I also did some follow-up interviews.

Through the 1980s most of the readiness commands had been holding annual weekend meetings of their medical departments in total, or at least the Navy Nurse Corps. Of course, you have to do some planning ahead in time for some of those conferences and what the programs are going to be. The Texas Fleet Hospital and Readiness Command were going to plan the conference at the end of the war. It was anticipated that most of the people in that fleet hospital had been mobilized. There were about 100 that had been mobilized to a variety of commands: a few to hospital ships, Marine detachments, etc. It was anticipated that those people would be back. I was to give the keynote address for their conference. This was the annual conference of nurses and corpsmen. The topic of the keynote was to be readjusting back home after being deployed. When I arrived, the surprise was that only one person had returned. I thought, "Uh-oh."

In talking to a few folks Friday evening, it was clear to me that the problems of readjustment after the war were also significant for those who were not deployed or mobilized from the reserve to any platform within the United States. I gave exactly the same speech, only it was about readjustment after not being deployed. What I didn't realize until five minutes into speaking is how deep those problems and feelings were. I hadn't spoken more than five minutes and half the people in the room were tearful. There was such relief on the part of people that were not deployed. From that two-hour session, it was very clear that we needed to have a debriefing experience for everyone in the Navy Nurse Corps in the medical department. We sent out an invitation from my office to all the regions that we would bring out a team with a set program if they would devote a weekend drill on the regional level for their medical reserve personnel. About two-thirds of the readiness command responded that they realized that debriefing was needed. Over the next six to eight months, we did just that.

Basically what happened, all that we asked the readiness command to do was to have a certain number of rooms reserved in one location for the conference and to identify people within their reserve components that who had had debriefing experience, whether they were counselors, psychologist, or psychiatrists, who had experience helping people adjust after traumatic events. Every Readiness Command had eight or ten such individuals.

I brought Jan Allen with me (one of the three reservists that we had mobilized by name), who was a very experienced in debriefing and counseling in the Veteran's Administration. She had been working in a large program for Vietnam veterans. On those conference weekends we arrived Friday afternoon with the group leading on Friday evening go over the schedule for the weekend. Jan would then have a training session with the debriefers. In other words, she trained the trainers. They were to be the group leaders for the weekend.

The weekend basically went like this: We had the whole group together whether it was 100 or 200 people. Jan and I alternated, but we went over the content of the first step in the process of debriefing. After we did that for about a half hour, they broke into groups. They broke up into groups with their group leaders to discuss and verbalize their feelings, experiences and thoughts about that piece of the process. They were broken up into groups according their experience during the war; mobilized to backfill a fleet hospital, with a Marine unit, on a hospital ship, or other small miscellaneous platform. The people that were not mobilized were also grouped together. They all had problems in common whether they were enlisted or officers. The groups were no bigger than about 15 people. If it was a large group, for example, if a readiness command had 150 people that went to a hospital ship, needless to say that was not one group.

That took about half the morning. Then we would get them back together to go through the next step. After that they would have another group session. They had four to six times together listening to the information as one big group and then breaking up to discuss that piece of the debriefing process.

When I went out to the Comfort, it was very clear that there were issues in interviewing people that had sailed back with the ship versus talking to people who had flown back to the United States. I was in Washington D.C. to welcome people who flew back to Bethesda. It was very clear to me that the people that sailed back had an easier adjustment back home than the people that flew home. The people that flew home from the war had a very sudden change in their environment and the people surrounding them, so they just didn't have a chance to adjust. The people that sailed back had much more time to talk with each other, to have time to themselves, time to walk, meditate, think and adjust to coming home. There were sessions on the Comfort for everyone before they left to prepare them somewhat for the changes and how to have a smoother emotional, mental, physical adjustment back home. For some it worked well; for others it didn't. I received a number of calls in my office from reserve Nurse Corps officers who volunteered to stay longer where they were mobilized, whether it was a hospital in the United States or in Saudi Arabia or Bahrain. There were some lingering overlapping needs for them to stay, and when volunteers were asked for, they'd call me and say, "I am staying a little longer. If you are communicating with my family, please don't tell them I volunteered, I don't want them to be angry with me. I need a little more time to adjust to coming back home." That was an interesting lesson learned.

Instead of staying for two years, Admiral Hall asked me to stay throughout her tour. That was four years, which included Desert Storm. She asked me if I would stay for a fifth year as a carryover person, because all the other active duty people in the office were leaving. I was at BUMED from September 1987 to September 1992.

There was interesting politics going on because Admiral Hall made it known I was to stay on active duty if I wanted to. I was too old to augment to USN when I came back on active duty so I was still classified as USNR. I got orders to go to Portsmouth Naval Hospital as the assistant director of nursing.

In May of 1999 I retired with events over a five day period. Many of my friends and colleagues came, which was heartwarming for me. The end of this month marks my six year post–retirement. That means that at the end of this month I am no longer eligible for mobilization or recall. For six years after one retires from the Navy, from reserve or active duty, you are on a recall list. The Army Nurse Corps recalled 50 of their most senior people, who had retired in the prior five years, back into positions they were in before they retired at the beginning of Desert Storm, before they looked at their reserve resources. The Navy would have been smart to do the same thing, to release some of the senior people to go where they needed to go, but have experienced people in their positions.

Totally, I had a three-stage retirement. I retired from the Navy in May 1999, I completed my term as president of Navy Nurse Corps Association in May 2000, and I retired from Old Dominion University in May of 2001. It was a step-wise retirement process. In the spring of 2001, when Iraq was invaded, the director of the Navy Nurse Corps Office received many calls from reserve nurses volunteering. They had to set up a phone number at BUPERS to identify what information they wanted from people. Within two weeks, over 200 Navy reserve nurses volunteered and had submitted that information, in case they were needed. I think that was a true testimony to that group.

Nancy L. Caldwell

Over nearly 30 years of nursing in the United States Air Force Nurse Corps, Nancy Caldwell did everything from working on the wards, operating room orthopedics, and obstetrics to being a chief nurse. She had been stationed at several duty stations in the United States as well as Japan, Greenland, and England. Finally, she got an assignment to Germany, a career-long desire. As an extra added surprise bonus, she also found herself pulling together all the experience she had and all the knowledge she had gained to make major decisions that impacted patient care during the first Gulf War.

I never thought that I wanted to be a nurse. However, by the time I was a teenager, I believe I was called by God to go into nursing. I felt such a strong need to do that. By the time I was a senior in high school, I could hardly wait to finish that year so that I could get on with nursing school. I felt such a strong sense that God put me where he did so that I could pursue a career in nursing. After graduating from a diploma school of nursing, Sparks School of Nursing in Fort Smith, Arkansas, and working in the private sector for several years, in 1963 I joined the Air Force. I chose the Air Force because John Kennedy had said we were going to the moon, and my friends and I were sure that the first woman to go to the moon had to be a nurse. There also was the opportunity in those days for nurses to get assigned to Patrick Air Force Base next to Cape Canaveral. We had two nurses assigned to the research team there. Also, we had nurses flying aeromedical evacuation, and that was another big draw to the Air Force. I thought that maybe that was something I could do. Besides, I didn't like the color of the other service's uniforms.

One day I got a telephone call from our assignments person. He said, "The general is going to call you. This is what she is going to ask you. Do you want to go to Europe to be the command nurse?" I had been waiting for years to get my Germany assignment. I said okay and quickly called my husband and said, "Do you want to go to Germany?" When the general called me and asked if I wanted the job, I said, "Yes, I would like to have it." I was thinking, "Oh, this is going to be a piece of cake. I already have this command nurse stuff down pat. I know how to get organized. I know what I have to do. I should be able to do this stuff without too much hassle. I will go over there, and I will have lot of time to sight-see and I will have a good time."

I went to Germany on the 22nd of July 1990 to be the command nurse for United States Air Forces in Europe (USAFE). On August 2 Iraq invaded Kuwait. I had thought that the only things I had to learn in Germany that would be different were where the bases are and where our wartime resources were. It turned out I had to be really speedy about learning that. The command in Europe at the time was a very big command. We had lots of clinics and hospitals. We had seven hospitals and 14 free-standing clinics. They were located all over Europe, Turkey and Spain. We also had eight large contingency hospitals. These were hospitals that were designed to be opened up to support the American troops in the event of a ground war in Europe.

As we were gearing up for Desert Storm, none of us initially knew exactly what we were going to be involved in or what was going to happen. We'd watch CNN to get our news. We were trying to figure out what we had to do to get ready. We decided at headquarters that even though we didn't know exactly what was going to happen, we would start expand-

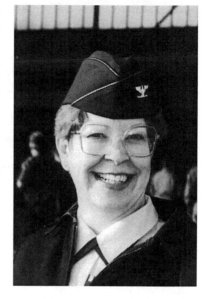

Nancy Caldwell filled the role of command nurse for the United States Air Forces in Europe (USAFE) from July 1990 until her retirement in November 1993. As a result she was in place to help orchestrate the movement of Air Force medical personnel for Desert Storm/Desert Shield. This picture was taken at Ramstein Air Force Base in 1991, at the end of Desert Storm/Desert Shield.

ing our hospitals and setting up aeromedical staging flights at places where we knew we would have groups of patients needing to be evacuated. Then we started looking at what we were going to do about our contingency hospitals because we didn't have any clinical staff assigned to them. They only had administrative staff to take care of inventory and maintenance. We decided initially that we would set up one contingency hospital at Zweibrucken, Germany, near the French border.

At Zweibrucken we had a building that had originally been a hospital. We put together a team from different bases that would go down there and get this hospital set up. I think we sent down 12 of them, and they worked day and night getting it ready because they had to start from the top floor down and clean everything. They had to take the beds out of the cartons and put them together. They had to take all the instruments that were packed in cosmoline (a petroleum-based compound the military uses to pack firearms and surgical instruments) and clean all that off before they could set up the instrument packs. They worked for two weeks, and it was amazing what they did. They set up the units. They set up an operating room so that it was ready to start processing instruments and handle patients. They set up the PACU and ICU. They had figured out what the patient placement and flow would be and how they were going to maintain safety. It was really pretty incredible what they did in two weeks.

I felt so very close to the situation in Iraq because the first fighter planes that went to Iraq were out of the First Tactical Fighter Wing at Langley Air Force Base, and they sent their air transportable hospital (ATH) along. So, I knew these people who were going out there. I was very glad that I had helped the ATHs to standardize things. My former boss said, "You know when those fighters show up with their air transportable hospital right behind them, they're not going to do an air show." We ended up having a lot of personnel from Tactical Air Command going over to the desert to do the fighting and provide medical care.

We continued to build up operations in Germany. We had to wait for the Air Force to tell us about personnel and supplies. We eventually opened up a total of seven contingency hospitals. We sent one of the nurses, a nurse practitioner, who had been a key player when the airplane fell out of the sky during an air show at Ramstein Air Base. She was a remarkable and well organized nurse. We sent her over to the Denmark to work with the Danes in setting up a contingency hospital there. Then we set up three contingency hospitals in England and a second in Germany. These were hospitals designed to support a war in Europe. But when we were supporting a war in Iraq, we knew that our patients would be coming from a lot further. We knew parents would be flying our direction if they knew their loved one was wounded and being aeromedically evacuated to Germany.

We also had to look at how we'd get our patients to the plane. We had to have an airfield for the plane to land and need to consider what resources we were going to need to get them to the contingency hospital. Sometimes it might be more than an hour by winding English roads from the airplane to the hospital. You had litter patients and now you were going to deal with patients with an increase in pain levels and nausea. So, there were lots of things to consider in caring for the war casualties.

In Germany we had the Germans coming out of the woodwork wanting to donate blood. We didn't accept their blood for our troops because we didn't know their immunization history. With our military donors we knew all the shots that they've had and what to screen for. So, we could be screening for something that could be significant. We had to tell these people no. That was very hard for them to accept. We had all kinds of people who wanted to volunteer. We had to figure out how we were going to use these volunteers in a way that was acceptable and that they would feel appreciated while protecting the patients and avoiding chaos. We had an aeromedical staging flight set up in Ramstein in a hanger and another at Rhein-Mein Air Base near Frankfurt. Eventually we had a hundred cots set up at Ramstein. We would sort the patients out there. Eventually, the Army patients would go over to the Army hospital at Landstuhl. The patients at Rhein-Main went to our Air Force Medical Center at Wiesbaden. Some would be put on the ambus (bus configured for stretchers) and sent down to that hospital in Zweibrucken that we set up.

We had to look at big flights. We would need additional manpower to manage all of the patients. If we are going to allow volunteers in the area, how do we control access and identify that they are trained volunteers? How do we make out schedules? These were all things that were different than anything we had faced before. Fortunately, the European representative to the Red Cross was an excellent nurse. She and I worked together to work out some of those things. As it ended up, we did not have the patient load that we thought we were going to have because the war was over faster than we thought it would be. It was very fortunate. But, if we had gotten the patients we thought we were going to get, we would have needed every last body.

When we originally set up these contingency hospitals, we knew we were going to need the help of the reserve forces. A lot of those reserves came in ones and twos, rather than a whole group. Once they got to Germany or England and had been in transit for two to three days, they were exhausted. Just because you have a surgeon doesn't mean you can have that surgeon working. You couldn't really get your hospital up and ready to go. You couldn't do those surgeries until you had your operating room contingent able to take care of PACU or ICU needs. So you might get most of your operating room contingent in, but not have an anesthesiologist or an anesthetist. We had to do a lot of communicating with our hospitals for them to be able to tell us that they would be ready to go and would be able to start accepting patients.

In wartime, all the aero medical evacuation teams came under the command of our headquarters. Ordinarily, they would have been under a different command, Military Airlift Command. But, in a time of war in Europe, the function of medical evacuation came under our command. So, not only were we supervising our facilities, but we were picking up aero evac, because we needed to be able to regulate where we were sending patients according to where we had beds and staff. It really was not an issue because the war was over before the ground war caused a lot of damage.

We haven't continued to use some of the plans we had in Desert Storm in Iraqi Freedom because of two things. One is after the Berlin Wall came down, we got rid of all the resources in those contingency hospitals. Maybe two were left. We dispersed that equipment to needy countries. The second thing is that they have rethought how they do the air transportable hospitals. They needed so much airlift to be able to transport them. They knew they needed to go to a system that was lighter and a lot more mobile. They have changed now to a concept of a team of six or eight with a surgeon and transport them very quickly. They are using some of the air staging principles. They are sending quite a number of the patients to Landstuhl. They have hospitals set up in Iraq for the current conflict.

We got through Desert Storm without as many casualties as we thought we would have. We had so many medical personnel deployed to Germany and England, but I don't know exactly how many there were. Wilford Hall is our big hospital in San Antonio. We had about 250 people from Wilford Hall or maybe it was 500. By the time we got all those people in and were trying to count noses, they were sending them home again. It certainly says a lot for our medical personnel, that we can be as flexible and innovative as we are to get things done. It never ceases to amaze me what people can come up with. One of the things we were faced with when we were doing this in Germany was that we would get all these people who had been trained in the ambuses in how to load, move, and turn and everything. Then they would get over to England and the doors were on the opposite side of the vehicles because they drive on the other side of the road. So, you had to think about what kind of training you were going to have to do for everyone so that they could work efficiently. Little things make such a difference. It is all those little things that nurses and med techs take into account when we are providing care. We are the ones that pay attention to the details.

I retired in November 1993 out of Europe. That was my 30 years. I thought I was retiring from nursing. I came back to the U.S. As I had traveled around the world, I had managed to get a master's degree from the University of Oklahoma. This was before the days of online educational opportunities. They had classes arranged around the missile officers in Minot when I was there. I started the master's program there. They would bring the instructors and professors in. When I was in Japan I could have gone to classes in Korea, but they didn't have anything I could use. So, I used self-study and independent study. Then, I went to MacDill. I had so much time and money invested in this, but the best place I could go to class was at the Pentagon. So, I would fly up and take a few days and go to the Pentagon. I would tell people that I was going to take classes at the Pentagon. They always thought I was going to the Pentagon for some very important business, and I just let them think it. When I went to Scott Air Force Base, I took my last class and did my comprehensives. My degree was in communications.

I always wanted a degree in nursing, so when I came back from Europe, I went to the University of Wisconsin School of Nursing at Madison. In 1997 I got a master's in psychiatric/mental health nursing as a clinical nurse specialist. In Wisconsin the role of mental health nurse practitioner is called clinical nurse specialist. I was going to market myself as a clinical nurse specialist when the job as the nurse administrator at a rural hospital about 23 miles from me came open. I had felt a very strong need to give back to the rural community. Good health care if you're having a heart attack or a baby is as important in the rural community as in the city. I took that job and in that position, I really took advantage of all that I had learned in the military to be able to do classes and help them move up to a different level in their management. I did that for five years until they about wore me out. Then for three years I worked intermittently for them, a little PRN working as nursing supervisor and helping them in writing grants. I had never written grants before,

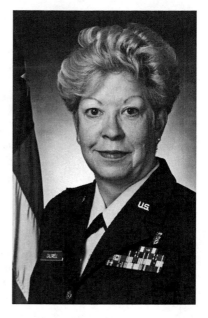

Nancy Caldwell at retirement in 1993.

but you know how it is in the military. You learn how to do things that you have never done before. I am still doing that job and will probably do it until early next year. Then I am going to quit altogether I think. It is time to do something different, time to spend more time with my husband. We are both 65. My family members live to be very old, but his does not, so I better spend some time with him while I can. We are going to travel. We have been traveling every year. We are going to travel to places we have never been before or to see friends we have all along the way. I think this year we are going back to Iceland. I have a nurse friend there. She came here last year, and now it's time for us to go and visit her.

I am very proud of my 30 years as a military nurse, though I feel my service pales in comparison to my colleagues whose stories are now being written.

MARIA CERRATO

Maria Cerrato tells of her experience in Iraq, of how much she learned and how much she was able to contribute because of her previous nursing experience. Because of her ability to synthesize the knowledge from previous nursing experience and apply it to her current situation in Iraq, she was able to make the decisions that contributed to better patient care and personnel safety. Maria's Gulf experience also opened up new opportunities for her to grow and expand in her professional and personal life.

I originally got a degree in liberal arts and worked as a social worker in Manhattan. Once I got married and had my first child, I decided to go back to nursing school. I did that after I had my second child in 1995. I was 27 years old. I graduated in 1998. I was pregnant with our third child, a son, at that time. I graduated from Sisters of Charity School of Nursing in Staten Island, New York. I decided to change to nursing because I felt that my time would more flexible with the children, and it turns out that is true.

I grew up in New York City, and I saw that all the hospitals in the area had a nursing shortage and figured that the Army would have one, too. So, after 9/11 I decided to join the Army reserve. I was 35 years old. The Army helped pay for some of my student loans and I got a sign-on bonus. I was doing the one weekend a month, two weeks a year thing when I was mobilized.

I got orders to report to Fort Sam Houston on November 22, 2004. It was after Desert Storm and already into Iraqi Freedom. It wasn't a surprise. I already knew it was a possibility. They were looking for people to go with the 228th Combat Support Hospital (CSH). I am from the 48th CSH out of Fort Meade, Maryland. I got cross-leveled to the 228th CSH. I volunteered to go. I figured I was going to go anyway, and I kind of wanted to control when it would be. My family was okay with me volunteering. They knew we would have a steady income, so that wasn't an issue. My boys were older. Jason was 12, Sean was 10, and Brandon was 7. They understood my role as a soldier, and my parents were a big support. I have been divorced for the last four years and was divorced when I was mobilized. The 48th CSH is presently slotted to go to Afghanistan again, and I will eventually be mobilizable again. I am in school full time right now, so maybe I won't have to go again for a while.

At the time I just wanted to get it out of the way. The timing was right. The kids were okay in school. My parents were with me and could take care of my children while I was gone. My daughter was still real young. Emily was only two years old.

I came to Fort Sam Houston from the Maryland area in November 2004 for a month of orientation, training, and paper work. We left the day after Christmas. I was happy they let us go home for Christmas, but we had to be back in the unit on Christmas Day. I went home to Maryland. This wasn't an easy thing. I was separated from my family. I was gone over the holidays. I did okay, though. I spent Thanksgiving in Texas, Christmas in Maryland, and New Year's in Kuwait. The hardest part was not knowing any of the people I was mobilized with. I was alone during my time in Fort Sam Houston.

Five hundred of us flew on commercial planes to Kuwait on two separate days. We were divided into two missions; one to Mosul and another to Tikrit. We stopped in Germany to refuel and landed in Kuwait early in the morning. The flight was pretty much a 24-hour flight. We landed in Kuwait so there was less concern about snipers or being attacked. However, we still traveled in the buses with curtains and we weren't allowed to open the curtains. I am not sure about the reason for the curtains. They had to have known there were soldiers aboard these buses. We had an American escort from the airport to the base, troops in trucks that traveled along beside us.

Kuwait is the area where everyone gets processed. We had to swipe our ID card to say that we were now in a combat zone. ID cards now are kind of digitalized in that they have a gold chip on them and a credit card strip. When you swiped it, they knew you were in country. We stayed at Camp Virginia. We all lived in tents, about 30 women to a tent, both officer and enlisted. It was not coed. I understand that in Afghanistan sometimes they live in coed tents. Sometimes there aren't enough tents. In Iraq the housing was separate. There were computers for us to use and there was a coffee station, kind of like a Starbucks. We could use the phones at the AT&T center, but you had to wait and you had to have a calling card. I didn't use the phone often, but I did use e-mail. Even e-mail was slow because a lot of people were using it.

I didn't really like Kuwait. It was sandy and when it rained it was just awful. We had running showers, but they were combat showers. That means that you get in the shower, turn on the water, turn it off, shampoo, and rinse off. You could do it every day, but it was kind of a trek to get to those trailers and we weren't sure when we would be leaving. It depended on whenever we were able to get a flight. It was a trek to the chow hall. It was a big base. There were Australians, Koreans, and other American units there. Everybody got shipped out from there to wherever we had to go. Each country processed its own people.

We left Kuwait shortly after New Year's. All the traveling was done in the middle of the night. They brought us to our destined forward operating base (FOB) by C-130, a little old plane. I hate flying on a C-130. They are uncomfortable. They pack you in like sardines. You can't move. They tend to use C-130s to get you from base to base or from FOB to FOB. We were stationed at FOB Diamondback. The C-130 isn't a quieter plane, but it is an older plane that kind of glides if it has to and you can't really see it at night.

When we left Kuwait we landed in Mosul, Iraq, at one o'clock in the morning. At this point I was like: "What am I doing here?" We had to get our gear. I had five full duffel bags and I was tired of carrying them around. They didn't expect us to come that late. We had to find rooms. They knew we were coming, but not exactly when. FOB Diamondback was right near an airfield to make off-loading patients easier. We landed in pitch dark, and it was a little chilly at that time of the year. There was a moon, but it was still so dark that you couldn't see your hand in front of your face. I guess we are so used to the street lights and living close to cities.

They got us situated. Some of us had rooms. Some had to sleep in tents. I had a nice comfortable room, though I shared with another person. If you were an E7 and above or a major and above, you had your own room. The living conditions were actually not bad. If I had had to go to Iraq in the beginning of the war, I probably would not have been able to make it the whole year. Living in tents, sleeping on cots, people walking in and out, not having hot showers—I don't think I could have done it. Nowadays everybody lives in a trailer. They were like the trailers construction people use when they are setting up a site. Each trailer had two dressers, air-conditioning, and a comfortable twin bed. I ended up getting a microwave, refrigerator, and a DVD player. It is comparable to living in a college dorm. Sometimes some of the units that were leaving would sell some of their things. The PX would sell some things like DVDs, TVs, and radios. There were also local people selling stuff on the base. We lived right next to the hospital, so we didn't have to walk very far. I have to admit I was pretty comfortable.

I am pretty outgoing and I knew pretty much everybody on the FOB. I just make friends easily. Two other girls and I kind of hung out together, and everybody would see us together all the time. They called us "the sisters." We didn't know each other before we got to Iraq. I got to know a lot of people.

I speak a Filipino dialect and so did my friends. Also, many Filipinos will float around working wherever they can, such as Saudi Arabia and Kuwait. So, there were a lot of Filipinos that took jobs in the alteration shops and as hairdressers and/or barbers. Some even worked as cooks in the chow hall, so I was able to eat my own food. Being around my people and eating Filipino food made my tour tolerable and closer to home.

My parents were the first generation to come from the Philippines in my family. My friends in Iraq were in sort of the same situation, though they were a lot younger, like 22 or 23. They had just finished nursing school and had been in ROTC while they were in school. They were brand-new nurses.

I worked in the ICU in Iraq. We only had ICU, ICW, which was like a step-down and regular ward combined, the ER, the OR, and the specialty clinic. When we got there we had to get oriented to the hospital, what to do, and how to do the paperwork. The unit we replaced wasn't very busy at that time, except for the big chow hall bombing in December 2004. That was their major event. During their tour, they were in tents and helped build the hardened facilities that we had. They were constantly being bombed and mortared. So, I have to hand it to them that they were able to get this fixed facility by the time we came in.

One of the major contractors in Iraq was KBR, an affiliate of Haliburton Corporation. They provided the Iraqi contractors to help build the hospital and other sites on the FOB. They are also responsible for delivering the food, the equipment, supplies for the PX, and all kinds of stuff. They even have their own convoy and security team.

As soon as the other unit left, we had our first MASCAL, or mass casualty. It went on sporadically from January 2005 until November 2005. I still talk to the people that replaced us, and they said that they still get just bits and pieces. I noticed that the amount of bombings decreased on our FOB once the new task force commander took control in April. Striker vehicles would go out and try and catch people that were trying to set off bombs or hiding the mortars or things like that. I think they had better control of communication with the police. Prior to that I think their mission was different. When we first got there, you could hear the mortars going off day and night. After a while I got used to it and just slept through it. They didn't have a specific target. They were just trying to hit whatever they could on the base. It was a big airfield with a prison, post–exchange, MWR and a movie theater.

There was a huge difference between then and 2002–2003. I had friends who went in 2003, and they tell how they had to use the same insulin syringes over again because they didn't have enough of them. They would have to recap and use them over again for the same patient. They would have to use the same bedpan for several patients. Everything was in tents. We didn't have that much of a problem. Our equipment was always there. We got supplied. Maybe there was one time when we ran out of fluid or IV tubing.

MASCALs are graded into level one and level two. Level one is 10–12 patients. Anything over 15 is a level two. The first MASCAL that we had was a level one that involved some children. We didn't have enough equipment for children. Our military vans (MILVANS) that carried our pediatric supplies had not arrived in Mosul yet. We had the wrong ET tube for children, as we soon learned with one of the children who came out of surgery and began having respiratory problems. We also found out that we didn't have any pediatric nurses. Aside from one PICU nurse, I had some experience with it. I was in charge during our next MASCAL, and I began assigning some nurses pediatric patients. It was do or die. They won't get over their fear if they don't just do it. So I told my friend that he would be taking the next pediatric patient. I told him I wasn't going to let him handle it on his own. It turned out to be the kid with the respiratory problems. He kept saying, "I'm going to kill this kid." I kept telling him, "I'm right here." As it turned out, we just needed to change the ET tube. We didn't even have a suction catheter that would go down the ET tube. We found one and we had to be careful not to throw it out because it was the only one we had.

In the beginning we had a lot of Iraqi soldiers, a lot of accidents and accidental shootings. It came in waves from Iraqi soldiers, Iraqi civilians and American soldiers. The American soldiers kind of tapered off by the end of the year. It became more of the Iraqi nationals. We also saw a lot of insurgents and POWs. We took care of them, just like everyone else. We actually had one that we knew was involved with the MASCAL that we took care of, but there wasn't enough evidence, so we had to let him go.

We saw a lot of traumatic amputations and IED burns. We had to make our own ISR (U.S. Army Institute of Research Brooke Army Medical Center) boxes. These were made of large cardboard boxes, and we used a bear hugger hose into the box to blow warm air around the patient to keep him warm and dry. Burn patients are just constantly seeping. The ISR box is part of the burn research being done at BAMC, Brook Army Medical Center.

We took care of a couple of contractors who were having acute MIs. One was a Turkish man that we actually saved and managed to get him to a Turkish Hospital. We had to send a Turkish doctor and nurse to fly this man back to Turkey. I had to train them on how to use our equipment; our pumps and our monitors. The patient made it. We also had a U.S. contractor who managed to get back to the United States. Both times I was off, but I just happened to be walking through the unit. We kind of liked to hang around the hospital during our time off. It wasn't like there was anywhere else to go. I am an open heart nurse. For one of these men, the ICU doc yelled at me, "Maria, quick!" One of these men was actually having the heart attack. You could see the EKG spikes. We shocked him and gave him lidocaine and he converted, so we started a lidocaine drip. The Turkish guy was a young guy. He was trying to climb out of the bed. He was going into V-tach and V-fib. They were trying to intubate him, and I yelled, "He's still awake." We were all on the bed and someone was going to shock him, and I had to stop them because we weren't clear of the bed. As you can imagine, things can get chaotic, especially with new nurses around.

I remember another incident with an Iraqi civilian. He had gunshots to his head. He had brain matter coming out of his nose and his skull was kind of partially off. He was bleeding everywhere. They were trying to sew him up. I had to say, "There is no way this man is going to make it. We just have to let him go." Finally, they agreed to let him go and gave him morphine. It really hit me that with his death someone needed to say something or say a prayer. Someone said, "Well, he's Iraqi." I said, "It doesn't matter." One of our ICU nurses is a minister at home, so he said a general prayer for him. It is interesting that the Iraqis don't have some sort of spiritual counseling there for their own people. There are a lot of Christians up in Mosul, and we didn't know if he was Christian or not. One of our interpreters was Christian.

Our last month there was Ramadan. We thought we would probably get a lot of hits. Two days in a row we got hit with a MASCAL. We were just overwhelmed and tired. It was one patient right after the other. They were all ICU patients; some kids and one fellow who was really injured with a chest wound. He had chest tubes and was on Levophed. We just felt he was going to die. He ended up making it. He stayed with us for a little while. He was the last patient in our ICU before we left. He was Iraqi so there was nowhere for him to go.

Once they were off the ventilator, we would send them to the Iraqi hospital. A lot of them didn't want to go because they knew they weren't going to get the same kind of treatment. They had to pay for pain medication up front. We would tell the patient that we were going to give them something for pain, and they would say, "But I don't have any money." We would say, "You don't need money." There are no nurses in Iraqi hospitals. There are just technicians who do all the care and administer the medications. The physicians came in the morning.

Some care was very difficult with the Iraqi patients because of the language barrier. For instance, it was difficult to get them out of bed or to have them turn, cough, and deep breathe, even with the interpreters. A lot of our patients were male, and they don't have a very high regard for women anyway. So, a lot of the men refused. They would do that hand signal that meant "go away." I would have to say to them, "Look, I'm not Iraqi. I'm not going away. You can't do that. You have to get out of bed and turn, cough, and deep breath." Some would respond. They would be able to tell that they were getting better, and they would tell the interpreter that they appreciated my care. Even the little boys treated women this way. They would be treating their mothers this way, by pushing them away or telling them to get out of their face. If they didn't want to do it, they weren't going to do it.

We did take care of a couple of women. One was miscarrying and on her way to the Iraqi hospital. There was a gunfight and she got caught in the middle. It was interesting because we didn't think about taking care of OB-GYN patients. I was an ICU nurse. We had to really think about having to monitor things like her bleeding and checking her fundus and things like that. We would comment, "Oh yah, I remember this from nursing." It was great because it was a lot of teaching and collaborating.

One patient had an abdomen that was getting hard. I said, "Why don't we do a bladder pressure?" "Can we do that here?" "Yes, we can. We have set ups for A-lines. It is the same thing." One fellow had a bladder pressure of 38. The docs said, "Forget the OR. Grab the stuff. We are going to do it right here." I knew that a normal bladder pressure is 18–25 from working in ICU. We do a lot of bladder pressures in ICU when you notice that they're not urinating and they are starting to get hypertensive. You wonder if they are bleeding into their abdomen and you don't know. So, you check for a bladder pressure. On this guy they had to open his abdomen up right there. He had had chest surgery and was bleeding into his belly. The fluid buildup was pressing down on his bladder and he wasn't urinating. So, we needed to relieve the pressure of all the fluid building up. They opened him up and just put a dressing and left him open. We put a wound vac on later to try to control the fluid loss and help him heal.

Wound vacs are pretty advanced for so far away. If we had been there in 2003, we would have had nothing. But, now we have advanced equipment over there. We have total care beds. It is pretty amazing. I was trying to get a cardiac chair up there because we were supposed to be getting patients out of bed. We couldn't get it because we couldn't figure out how to order it with the right model and order number. So, we used lawn chairs, though they weren't very stable. We are now going to get PCA pumps, which are going to be universal throughout all the facilities. That way, when patients go from Iraq to Germany or to BAMC, they will just have to change the pumps out.

It seems we will be in Iraq for a while. The last I heard it was going to be 2010. They were discussing giving up the whole FOB in Mosul to the nationals. They were talking about moving us to a different facility. But, that hasn't happened yet.

I saw in the *Nursing Spectrum* that there is a nurse from some hospital that just finished graduating the first class of Iraqi nurses who are going to begin taking care of Iraqi patients. The nurse in charge is from some big hospital here in the United States. I think they graduated 20 nurses.

In Iraq there haven't been a lot of nurses, and a lot of the women weren't able to be nurses because of their culture. The culture requires that they be home at a certain time; family comes first. They aren't allowed to touch men that aren't their husbands or sons. Many of their resources were antiquated. There weren't enough books. We are collecting nursing books to give to them. This was a mission for one of the civil affairs units stationed in Iraq. They would go see what kind of hospital was needed and how to train personnel. Some of their medications they buy off the black market.

I came home in November. It was a commercial plane, and we stopped in Ireland for refueling and then landed in San Antonio. My family was not there to meet me because I wasn't sure exactly when I would come in. I didn't want them to have to fly over and take the kids out of school. I told them I would call when I got here. I didn't want to go through the welcoming thing. I was tired. We came, again, in the middle of the night. There was a big parade. I was like, "Okay, this sucks. My family isn't here. I just want to go home and sleep." We had to find our gear again, load up, and get to the barracks. We didn't get to bed until about two or three in the morning and then we had formation at 0530.

We landed Friday morning and they were rushing to try to get us all exited out. They wanted active duty people out and back to their own duty stations by Monday. They didn't have to do all the things that we did because their own duty stations could take care of any problems, like physicians or post–deployment stuff. As reservists, they were kind of up in the air. They weren't going to do anything. We asked, "What if we had issues in Iraq?" A lot of people were on medical hold. I was on med hold because when we first got to Iraq we had the old suction equipment. If you have a ward full of patients all on suction machines and wound vacs and all kinds of equipment, many of us went deaf. If you had a MASCAL with several patients on suction machines, it was pretty loud. Someone actually came in and tested the noise in the ICU and it was significant. They said, "If this continues, people are going to lose their hearing." We couldn't even hear each other in the unit. We wore ear plugs and we were always saying, "What?" So, I wanted someone to give me a hearing test when I got back to San Antonio. The test showed I had a little bit of hearing loss and now it is documented. Many people were in the same situation. The situation has gotten better because now they have quieter suction machines. That one thing, the possibility of hearing loss, made a difference in what kind of equipment we use.

I was at Fort Sam for almost a month, and I hadn't seen my family yet. So I decided that if any medical condition came up, I would deal with it later. There was so much red tape and people who couldn't decide whether they were supposed to do physical exams on reservists or not. I left there in December 2005, back to being a civilian and a reservist. I moved to San Antonio in July, and I just met a bunch of people who just got off med hold. They all had surgeries or medical issues, but they have been on active duty all this time because they are on med hold. I was lucky that my only issue was the hearing, and maybe I should have seen other physicians, but I just opted to not do that. I filed with the VA and I am supposed to have a five or 10 percent disability later on when I retire.

I got home right before Christmas. I signed my DD214 on Christmas Eve. I got through Christmas and went back to my job. Technically, you're supposed to have 90 days before you go back to work, but I was already off active duty. I wasn't getting a paycheck. So, I went back to work. I wasn't really okay with that. I needed the rest, but I needed the money. I was tired. I didn't want to see any more patients. I didn't want to suction anyone else. I needed the time off, but I couldn't do it, being the sole support for my family. I went back to the same unit I left at Walter Reed, where I work as a civilian.

My family was all excited about me coming home. They were very excited to see me, but I was so tired with the time change that I would be falling asleep at 8 P.M. We seemed to go back into the same routine. While I was in Iraq my father would call me or e-mail me with some issue, and I would be frustrated. I couldn't do anything. I was in Iraq. I would have my son scan and e-mail as much stuff as possible. Sometimes it would come okay, sometimes not. Then he would have to try again. I have an autistic child so there was a lot of paperwork involved with the doctor and appointments and those kinds of things. My parents could make some decisions, but not others. I was going through a child-support hearing at the time. They needed paperwork from me and some things had to be notarized. It is pretty amazing that we could even have scanning and e-mailing things as an option.

I have been home almost a year now. I think I'm doing okay. I don't think I have any symptoms of PTSD. It isn't in my nature to have any of that kind of thing. I am the oldest of four. I don't have time to get depressed. I have kids I have to take care and I am always on the run. My parents still live with me. They have always been around to take care of my kids while I was working and going to school. They helped my kids grow up and my kids are used to having their grandparents discipline them.

I moved from Maryland to Texas. The people in the 228th CSH were from Texas, and they kept telling me how nice it was in San Antonio. They said how family friendly it was. I was kind of getting tired of the East Coast with its fast pace, rude people, congestion and cold weather. I think I just wanted to get away from all that. I wanted to buy a house, and I couldn't afford to do that in Maryland. My dad saved the money I made while I was in Iraq. We looked at some houses in Texas and found one big enough for my whole family.

I am anticipating going back to Iraq again. My son is autistic and there were a lot more services available to him while I was on active duty. The pediatrician took the initiative to start those services, like speech therapy. Now that I am working on my bachelor's degree, there is a 50 percent chance that I will go active duty. The health care benefits for my son were great. Once you become captain, the pay is pretty good. My pay while I was in Iraq was about equal to my civilian pay because they paid you combat pay, hazardous duty pay and housing. I was able to save some money while I was there. I like active duty pay because it is more regular, twice a month on the same dates instead of simply every other week.

There are lots of opportunities for me as part of the Army Nurse Corps. There are classes and schools like CRNA schools. I feel like a regular staff nurse. I'm not going anywhere. I have been a nurse in the ICU for the last six years, even though I have been a nurse for ten years. There isn't a lot of room for me to grow or expand. And if I wanted to change to education or research, they are always looking for experience. Right now I am working at BAMC. Most of the civilian hospitals in San Antonio are still doing paper charting. I'm not used to that. Computer charting saves me so much time. I can just click, click, click and go on to my patient. I don't have to flip through pages of information. I can just look on the computer.

Having been to Iraq and moving to San Antonio has opened more options for me and my career. I learned a great deal as an Army nurse. The reason why I became a nurse was exemplified ten fold as I took care of Iraqi and American soldiers. It is time for a career change. With the continued support of my family and God, I can now move on to another page in my life. Things happen for a reason. I am honored to serve my country and my patients.

PETER CHAREST

Many nurses have life experiences that enrich their nursing experience and the care they provide to their patients. Peter Charest took a rather circuitous route to nursing, but one that served himself, the military and his patients well. Peter came home from the war changed by his experiences, wiser and more sensitive, concerned about the impact of one's experiences on life, a more competent practitioner, a stronger leader, a better nurse.

I went into the Coast Guard in 1979. I was in the Coast Guard for 15 years. I was an EMT involved in law enforcement and search and rescue. I went to EMT school in Petaluma, California, for the Coast Guard in 1984. I was 24 at that time. I didn't go to college until 1987 because I was saving up money for the VEP Program, the Veterans Education Preference Program.

I came from Gloucester, Massachusetts, and grew up in the fishing industry. We didn't have a lot of money growing up. The military was the only way of my getting an education. I saved enough money after eight years of active duty that I decided to go into the United States Coast Guard reserves and go to college. On my days off, when I wasn't going to school, I drove ambulance in and around the Boston area. In 1991 I decided to go to nursing school. I was torn between going into criminal justice and nursing. Criminal justice was what I did in the Coast Guard as Coast Guard boarding officer and doing drug and fishery enforcement in New England.

Then I started working the ambulances and I really enjoyed it. Also, to put myself through nursing school, I worked as an emergency room technician at Salem Hospital in Salem, Massachusetts. I really loved doing EMT stuff. I was in college at Salem State in Massachusetts, part of Massachusetts State College, and I was kind of running out of my VEP money. I found out from Senator John Kerry that if you enlist in the military through Massachusetts, you are considered a state veteran and you get free tuition. I went back to school and continued in nursing at Salem State, which is considered one of the best-rated schools of nursing in the state. I got my BSN.

I had graduated in 1991 at age 31 from Salem State with a criminal justice degree. I graduated in 1994 with a BSN at the age of 34. I got into nursing because one day as I was leaving Salem State College, they were having this career day. This very attractive Navy Nurse Corps lieutenant named Tina

Nawrocki, now Commander Tina Ortiz stationed at Bethesda, said, "Oh, we can take you in the Navy Nurse Corps." I had been trying to get a commission in the Coast Guard and could never get one. I basically did a lateral transfer over from the Coast Guard to the Navy. I had had 15 years in the Coast Guard. I was over halfway to retirement. I came in the Navy as an ensign with 15 years of experience. I wasn't a junior officer. I was junior by rank, but I still had a lot of time behind me.

My first duty station was Naval Hospital San Diego, working on the wards and then in the operating room. I got transferred to Naval Hospital Okinawa, Japan, and was there for three and a half years working in the operating room. It is one of the biggest in the Pacific Rim. We only ran four rooms, but we averaged about 450 cases a month. That was the scheduled cases. We were the only ones that had orthopedic surgeons and we had two neurosurgeons. Anyone in the whole Pacific Rim would actually come to us first and we would medevac them out to Tripler, Hawaii, or back to the United States. Okinawa gave me a pretty broad experience as far as being an OR nurse. We saw a lot of trauma.

I got orders to Great Lakes Naval Hospital in July of 2002 to the OR. I have been an OR nurse since '96, so no matter where I go in the Navy, I am always going to work in the operating room. I am in charge of the OR here at Great Lakes. We have eight rooms, but we only run four of them.

I was deployed February 2004 through October 2004. I was with the First Marine Expeditionary Force in Fallujah, Iraq, during the initial storm of the city. The Marines went in and relieved the 782nd Army Division that had been there for 14 months. We were under General James T. Conway out of Camp Pendleton and we went into Fallujah, Iraq, and took the city back from the insurgents.

The experience was nothing like the war movies you grow up watching on TV. We came into the camp under fire. We had been dropped off in the middle of the night. We got fired on before we even got onto the ground. The National Guard helicopters were firing back. I was at a camp called the MEK, which was actually one of Sadam Hussein's training bases. He also used it as a terrorist training camp for the Iranians, who used to come in there and train, too. They knew the base. They knew the outline of the base. The base was only eight miles from the city of Fallujah, Iraq. They would hit all the time with incoming rocket mortar rounds. From the first day we got there, they were just throwing rounds at us all the time.

The most memorable thing that stands out is that every time we had a mass casualty drill, we ended up having the real thing come in. We were fired on the whole time we were doing surgery on people. I still have memories of the worst day we had. It was Saturday, March 20. At 0500 in the morning they were incoming us with mortar rounds. We got hit all day long. At eight o'clock at night two French-made 122 type rockets hit the back door of our hospital.

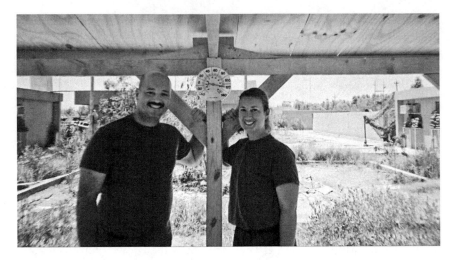

Peter Charest on his birthday, 17 July 2004 in Camp Al Fallujah, Fallujah, with an unidentified fellow soldier.

We were taking the turnover from the 782nd Army. One of the general surgeons and a medic got killed by the rockets. It actually blew the back door of our hospital off. It hit one of our corpsmen in the neck and injured six people. I weigh about 200 pounds in all my battle gear, and I was at the other end of the hospital, probably about 30 feet away, and the explosion knocked me down. The thing that really made me appreciate life was that about 20 minutes before that, I was in a warehouse where we kept all our supplies. I had walked through there carrying a case of normal saline. I had just gotten to the other end and put the normal saline up on the operating room floor when the rockets came down. If it had been 20 minutes earlier it would have been my time to go.

The surgeon was on the cell phone talking to his wife. There weren't enough pieces to pick him up. The medic got hit in the chest. His breast bone had a four-inch hole in it. When we rolled him over, the exit wound was bigger than a hubcap on a car. He talked to us. We ripped his clothes off. We didn't even put on sterile gear. We just poured betadine on his chest. We cracked his chest open and six inches of his aorta was gone. There was nothing we could do. I have never seen a man bleed out like he did. I think that was the hardest thing. I knew him and I was the nurse; I was his nurse. I was intubating him and putting him to sleep. I was one of the last individuals to ever hear anything come out of his mouth. There was just a river. I have never seen anybody bleed as fast as he did. It was like pouring buckets of water on the bed.

That first couple of weeks really bonded our surgical company together. From that day on it was like that every day. They woke us up or at night time shelling us. You didn't know if you went out to the Porta-John if it would be the last 15 seconds of your life. Every day was like March 20.

When the rockets fired the 122s, you could hear them whistle through the air. When you get used to it, you can kind of get a jump and start running for the nearest foxhole or seven-ton truck to duck under. The motors on the rockets are silent. They also have different ranges and sizes on them. Outside the base there was an automobile junkyard. The insurgents would hide in the junkyard and set up the mortar rounds. They would pack ice inside the tubes and then put the mortar inside the tube. By the time the ice melted in the 120 degree temperature, they would be long gone. By the time the Marines and the radar system would track them, there would be nothing there but the empty tube. You never hear them coming in. They are just silent and then all of a sudden, something explodes behind you.

You can't really trust anybody over there. I don't mean to sound prejudiced or anything. The press would go, "What about the little kids or the old ladies?" I got to tell you, those little seven- and eight-year-old kids are running armaments. They are the ones carrying the rocket reloads for the insurgents. The old ladies you think are nice people. You are driving down the street and they are waving to you. They have remote detonators just waiting for you to go a couple of feet up the road. All of a sudden there is an abandoned truck blocking you and the convoys are all backed up. Every 10 or 20 feet they bury these IEDs in the ground. There isn't just one. They stack them three or four deep. Then the trucks stop and all of a sudden all these explosions go down in sequence. The old lady who was waving to you and blowing you kisses is long gone and everything is on fire. You can't hear anything because the percussion has made you deaf. You are always looking over your shoulder. You don't really trust them.

We saw guys trying to shoot themselves in the foot. That was a common occurrence. We had guys that were in the latrine, and they would come in with a gunshot round to the foot because the gun went off accidentally as they were going to the bathroom.

The other big thing that I witnessed was that they wanted us to pull out of Fallujah, Iraq. We were supposed to win the hearts and minds of the citizens of Fallujah. The snipers were still up in the mosque towers and patrolling the outer perimeter of the city. For four or five days we kept getting guys coming in with sniper wounds to the head, face, and neck, and they were paralyzed from the neck down. These guys are 18, 19, 20 years old. We had guys coming in who had lost both legs and an arm, 21 years old. I'm thinking, "Well, you know, I can't really complain about what I've got."

Everybody in my company was great. We all pitched in. We did emergency work. We took bodies to the morgue. We did sandbagging. We all just pitched in, captains on down. We spent the first four days putting up the Texas barriers after the rocket attack. Texas barriers are like the Jersey barriers or road barriers. They are about 15 feet tall. They are big and you need a big crane to move them. They put those, like a protective barrier, all around our hospital and our berthing area. We just sandbagged everything else. From the captains on down, nobody complained. We just did what we had to do. It was a lot like MASH.

I can watch the MASH episodes now on TV, and I know the sleep deprivation. You don't know what time it is, even what day it is, after you have been in surgery for over 30 hours straight. You get out of surgery after 20 hours; lay down for 45 minutes before you have to go back into surgery again. You eat the things that people send you that you are so happy to see, like a box of crushed Oreos. You're just happy to see them, like a package of beef jerky. Sometimes we didn't get chow supplies. We would eat MREs and just drink lots of cheap Folgers's coffee and ate a lot of Pop-Tarts. I really appreciate now taking a hot shower, having clean clothes, not having to sit in the gravel and the dirt and worry about the scorpions and the camel spiders. I appreciate having a hot meal. I am very short on tolerance for people who complain that they don't have everything. My whole life has changed.

One of the big things in terms of the images I have is that being the officer in charge of the OR, I was also the officer in charge of the morgue. I had to tag and bag all the body parts and put them in the reefer. We all pitched in. We had a petty officer that was in charge of it, but as far as taking the body off the operating room table and bagging it up and collecting all the valuables and then physically taking the body from the operating room out to the morgue, I had to do that. We had to carry all the bodies out. Sometimes they wouldn't pick them up right away, so they would be stacked up in there from a couple of days. Then they would come and pick them up. I have that image of always opening up the back of the tractor trailer doors that was the morgue. That was pretty standard in the theater of operations. It had a little air-conditioning unit on the other side of it, so it was kind of like a reefer box. They would come with a seven ton and put the bodies in the back and then put them in a helicopter and fly them out from our base. I had to move the bodies from the operating room to the trailer-morgue. Then I would have to move them from the morgue to the helicopter because I had to account for the tag numbers to make sure nobody got left behind. I kept a spreadsheet of all our cases while I was in Iraq. As I look at that spreadsheet and all the names and numbers, I can remember them all and put a face back on them.

One guy I will never forget. He was a Seabee. His name was John. He was a chief. It was one of the toughest days we had. Some incoming mortars hit the Seabees' compound. We had two urgent surgeries and two killed, all medevaced to the CSH. It was one of the longest days we ever had in the operating room. John thought he was going to lose his leg. We did everything we could to save it. In an issue of *All Hands* magazine, there was a picture where he was actually standing up getting his Purple Heart award. We were very happy to see him standing on his two feet. When he left us, I didn't think he was going to make it. I thought he would lose his leg. He actually lived and is doing pretty well, I guess.

One time we had been mortared all day and all night. Towards dusk, a couple of jets went overhead, pretty close to the OR. A C-130 fixed-wing gunship came down and swooped over the camp. He circled around the base. Then about a mile and a half outside, over the wall, you just saw this big puff and heard his cannon fire. Then, you saw this big puff of orange smoke go up. He came over and locked on these Iraqis who were out setting up a little mortar tube in the junkyard. He did a little half circle, banked the plane and took them out.

On Saturday, September 11, I was in the warehouse and a rocket came down. It knocked the wind out of me. It knocked the wind out of one of our corpsmen. This is how it was until we left. They were just hitting us with mortar and rocket rounds every day.

One time I was out walking toward the shower trailers and two rockets came over. I started running and climbed underneath a seven-ton truck and laid there. They hit the ammo dump on our base that day and all the ammo that we had stored up was just flying around the base.

Two people that were with me in the Gulf in my company were John Seifert and George Merbetz. Seifert was an emergency room doctor, our trauma physician in the company. George was a podiatrist from California. When the Army left, they took their orthopedic surgeon with them. For a month and a half, we didn't have anybody but George. We just had the two general surgeons and George. They didn't give us an orthopedic surgeon. So, Captain Dana Covey had to fly down from another base and join our company. We just had too many orthopedic cases. He is the orthopedic specialty leader for the Navy. He had extensive deployments in Bosnia and Afghanistan. He is well-published, well-versed, and he has a lot of experience. We were glad he came and joined our company because we really needed him.

We didn't have tourniquet machines, part of standard equipment at naval hospitals. We only had field external fixation sets. When the Army left, they took their tourniquet machine. We were doing a lot of leg trauma and amputation cases and we had no way to stop the bleeding. When Dr. Covey got there, he backdoored and called a friend of his in Portsmouth. They shipped us, FedEx, two tourniquet machines and the large fixation sets. All we had was the standard field sets with one size of pins, but we never expected a lot of the civilian casualties, especially the little kids. None of these big-pin sets would do any good for them. He got the sets with various size pins sent to us to do the external fixations. I think we saved a lot of blood loss. We saved a lot of lives with his ingenuity of getting these machines to us.

I am surprised that in the AMAL system or the supply system for deployment, these machines, that are the size of a desktop computer screen, aren't standard equipment. I went to a medical conference in Bethesda, Maryland, in January 2006. The Medical Corps was there, and I explained to them that they needed to update these systems. It is not hard to pack two tourniquet machines. They are battery operated, and you can hook them into a generator, as well. It was very frustrating telling folks at the BUMED level about the needed updates. I still get e-mails from folks over there who have worked for me asking me to send them stuff through the Army supply system. We try to do that and have the materials FedEx led to them. I don't have to pay for the equipment, but I pay for the postage out of my pocket. It is faster if you FedEx it to Kuwait airport than if it goes through the government mail system. The military postal service will pick it up at Kuwait International Airport and bring it to whatever base it is addressed for.

I should talk about some of the patients we took care of. John came to our base in September. A rocket came down and hit the Seabee compound and John had fragment wounds to his right foot, left thigh and a nerve injury. Captain Covey operated on him and we shipped him out. Kent had an IED injury. An IED hit the Hummer he was in square on. The Hummer rolled over and took his left distal femur and his leg off.

We had one fellow named Shane. He was a civilian guy that runs those little remote control planes; those little spy planes that they fly over Fallujah, Iraq. That is how they see if the insurgents are running in and out of the different neighborhoods. A rocket came down and hit him. A piece of shrapnel went into his back, but instead of going straight into his rib cage, it deflected and went up underneath his skin, up by his shoulder blade. We took out a four by six piece of shrapnel, and he was actually very lucky to be alive. It was a posterior chest foreign body. All we did was take it out, wash him up, send him back to our recovery ward and then back to work.

I can't remember one gentleman's name, but he was actually one of the luckiest corporals I ever saw. He was wearing his flack vest, got hit by an AK-47 round. He was riding in a Hummer, the passenger on the right side, and they shot him through the door. Instead of going straight into his rib cage, it broke a piece off his Kevlar vest. The bullet deflected off the Kevlar, went underneath his skin, broke two of his ribs and went in the track of his rib cage and sat right on top of his chest under his skin. He was lying awake on our little trauma table, and you could see the bullet right there under his skin. They just cut it out right there and stitched the guy up. He ended up taking a indelible marker and writing Happy Birthday on his head. He was one of the luckiest people we ever met. The bullet was about three or four inches long. It was a big caliber round bullet. They sent him to the ward for a little bit and then they sent him back to his unit.

I'll always remember one July at midnight. The Marines are out patrolling, and this 70-year-old man was driving a car up to a checkpoint and he wouldn't stop. In the car with him was a little four-year-old Iraqi girl. We didn't know if the man was her father or grandfather, but they both came in with gunshot wounds. They were running the checkpoint and they wouldn't stop. She came in looking like a disheveled, dirty little four-year-old. What she was doing out at two o'clock in the morning with some 70-year-old guy, I have no idea. He was shot in the left forearm, left leg and left thigh, and she was shot in the left flank and the right forearm. We ended up doing a left flank evisceration.

We put a lot of hours in that night. On the left side of the child's stomach, all the intestines came out. We ended up doing an exploratory laparoscopy on her and small bowel repair. It was things like that that were so surprising. We weren't expecting to do a colostomy take down on a four-year-old. I'm thinking my son, Mattie, back home, is four years old, and I am trying to put myself in that place. The little girl survived. She ended up with an open iliac fracture. We ended up putting some pins in her hips and an external fixation set on her pelvis. She had an ulna fracture. Her bladder was nicked, which we fixed, and we put her bowel back together. She was tough little girl and she hung in there. We medevaced her up to Baghdad.

The older man survived and the Marines ended up taking him up to the custody hospital in Baghdad. That was like the prisoner-of-war section. It is the humanistic side of war like this case that kind of stays with you and you talk about them. For four days, every time we had breakfast or dinner we would talk about it. We just couldn't get any answers to exactly what happened. Sometimes there was a lot of confusion, too. We kept trying to figure out who was who and who belonged to whom. We had interpreters trying to talk to this particular Iraqi guy, and he wouldn't give us any information.

We actually operated on one of the police German Shepherds. He got his paw cut in some razor wire. We didn't have a vet. George did the nitrous and put the tendon back together. One of our nurse anesthetists put the dog to sleep. He started an IV on the dog. The lance corporal was there the whole time, and we kind of gave the dog conscious sedation so it wouldn't bite us. George repaired the paw and the dog was fine after that. He became our mascot dog. He would always come down to visit us.

We had an old Iraqi man who stayed with us for the longest time. He lost his lower leg. We thought he was an insurgent. For some reason, he was firing at the Marines and they shot him in the right leg. He ended up getting amputated. He would only eat MRE meals because he didn't trust us unless the food was in a package. We would escort him out to the port-a-john, but we couldn't understand why his leg kept getting infected or was continually staying infected. Every time he would go out to the port-a-john, he would take his bandage off and with all the flies there he would start picking at his wound. Finally, we caught on to what he was doing. He didn't want to go back to where he had come from. We fit him with a prosthetic and sent him away. He was with us for about three weeks. The prosthetic was an old prosthetic we had that looked like it had been left over from Vietnam. It was still pretty fancy for an Iraqi.

We had a lot of prisoners. We had a little prisoner-holding facility on our base. A lot of them had external fixations on their forearms from broken forearms or humeral fractures. They would have to come back every other day to have their dressings changed. They would always bring them in blindfolded and handcuffed. They didn't want them to know different areas of the base. It was very secretive. They stayed blindfolded during the transfer, but they would take off the blindfold while we treated them. We weren't worried about them seeing personnel, just the orientation of the base.

There was another guy called Carson. He was a Marine private. He was a frequent flyer. He came to us three separate times when he got injured. The third time they decided to ship him out of country. They shipped him out to Baghdad, then Germany and then back to Camp Pendleton.

Dolan and Frank were both corporal scout snipers with the 31st Marine Division. One day in July they were hit by rockets. Frank had multiple shrapnel wounds in his extremities and his trunk. He actually had fragments embedded up to his right quadriceps tendon. We could see them on X-ray, embedded in the muscle tissue of his thigh, but when we were trying to get them out we just couldn't remove the fragments. We removed what we could and hoped he didn't get infected and then medevaced them out. We kept picking these fragments out of his buttocks and we couldn't figure out what they were. Then we realized they were the Kevlar seating in his Humvee. The explosion blew those fragments up inside of him.

Bakri was a fuel truck driver that ran a road block. They shot him. That night he came in with a traumatic arthrotomy of the knee. Basically, he didn't have any knee left. He basically lost his whole knee joint, and we ended up doing a popliteal bypass on him. We put the gortex graft in to maintain the circulation in his leg, but he didn't have a knee left. We put him on the helicopter to Baghdad. So, this man ran a road block to hurt us. We shot him and then we had to fix him.

Ethically, as a nurse, I understood how the system went and how Captain Seifert wanted it. It was surgery, and whoever had the highest surgical priority went first. It is kind of tough to tell a Marine sergeant or captain why we are taking the bad guy who just killed two of his guys and wounded four others and tried to blow them up with a roadside fire bomb to surgery first, even though he was the bad guy. I didn't understand that part. In the military you have the ethics of being a naval officer, but then you have the ethics of being a nurse and the ethics of being a human being. If Captain Seifert tells me a guy needs to go to surgery first, then he needs to go to surgery. If I had been in the decision-making position, I would have done the same thing. You have conflict when you have bodies coming through the door and you have to tell the Marines that they have to wait. We almost came to blows with the Marines, them getting in my face and swearing at me. I had to say, "I understand what you are saying, but this is how we treat patients here. A bad guy or a good guy, whoever has to go first, goes first. I don't make the rules. I am just following the rules of surgery." I think that was one of hardest decisions, the ethical decisions of bad guy first and giving them all our blood and doing surgery on them and shipping them off.

They sent us an Army colonel who was an anesthesia doctor. I guess he and the Army had some different views about this ethical decision. He was just adamant all the time about doing this stuff. He wanted to treat our guys first. It made my life difficult because he's a colonel and I'm a lieutenant. But, it's like: "Sir, you know Captain Seifert is the director and he says this guy is going to surgery." "Crap, this isn't right. We got out own guys up there bleeding. Here I am working on this scum bag, this low life."

The decision on the part of the Iraqis to be there fighting was probably not their own. They were probably forced. We had a lot of innocent civilians caught in the cross fire of the insurgency. They were just kind of caught in the war zone.

Another guy we had was Assad. He was 27 years old. He also ran a checkpoint and the tank battalion hit his car on purpose. He came to us at six o'clock in the morning. This had happened at nighttime. He had shrapnel wound to the right tabula neck. He also had a right pulmonary contusion. He was a big hefty guy that we had lying face down and intubated with a big neck wound. They wanted to save this guy's life. He had killed four Marines at a checkpoint. He got shot in the neck, but the explosion blew him out of the truck. We ended up fixing this guy up and sending him up to the CASH (Casualty Army Surgical Hospital). He got medevaced. I don't know if he survived. He was just breathing when we got him.

Another gentleman I remember was Clyde. He was a first lieutenant, Marine Corps. It was early in the morning during a border attack in Ramadi. He had left leg shrapnel wounds with hemorrhage. He had a non–displaced left tibia fracture. The popliteal vein was lacerated. We ended up doing a bypass on him. It is amazing that we can do that on the front. Amazingly enough, with all the surgeries we did and all the flies that landed in the wound sites and the dust that we lived under, we had a very low infection rate, even with the harsh conditions we had to work under.

The question that frequently gets asked is: "Are we doing any good over there?" I am not sure we are doing anything. I am just very concerned that we are getting ourselves into something. I don't understand why the Iraqis aren't taking back their country yet or taking back the fight. I thought we were doing some good in the beginning, but now I am kind of questioning how long we have to be over there. I just don't see this thing ending any time soon. We are going to be there for the next five to ten years. My own experience in talking to the Marines is that they take the Iraqi Army guys out in Fallujah, Iraq, to patrol and as soon as they got into a fire fight, the Iraqis would throw down and run away. They would either scatter or they wouldn't fight. It took them a while to get them to fight and stick up for themselves. On the news, every time the Iraqis are going to take their country back, they are always saying they want us to stay. How long do you need to stay? I am having a hard time understanding why we are still there. When I look at the killed in action (KIA) numbers, they just keep climbing.

When I left the camp we got up at two in the morning. We wanted to go to Al Asad, which is the nearest air station. We were going to catch a C-130 out of Iraq back down to Kuwait. You have to go through the industrial center of Fallujah, Iraq, and that is eight miles straight across, but that is where they burn the guys on the bridge. They burn bodies off the bridge. So that is where you don't want to go. So, we had to take a convoy in the middle of the night 131 miles around, a half C, rather than the eight miles straight across.

The first mile outside the camp, the first hour, was the worst because that is where the insurgency is. We got ahold of the tank battalion on base, and they gave us an escort through the overpasses to make sure that our 30-member convoy got out safely. Then we had two of the trucks break down and they started hitting us with mortar rounds. We just climbed on somebody else's truck. We got down to Al Asad. The truck I was on didn't break down, but when you are kind of sitting out there in the sand dunes in the middle of the night it is not a good thing. It doesn't take anything for them to pop up over a sand dune.

The loud noises are the scariest things I found when I came back, even when I was walking up the walk to the supermarket with my kids. I had them in a jogging stroller. They were doing some roofing in the house across the street. The guy is using a pneumatic nail gun, and I thought somebody was sniper firing at me. I was going back behind the hedge at my neighbor's house and my sons are going, "What are you doing, Dad?" If the trash guys come and they take the big dumpster and they empty it and they bang it down on the ground, I think it is like a mortar round coming in. I get real jumpy. It took me a while to get used to being home. It was surreal. It was like everything was different. It was like it wasn't my life anymore. My whole life was changed, my house and my kids. I don't think I will ever be the same.

I have a little post–traumatic stress going on that I am getting seen for. I'm always looking over my shoulder. I am always leery of people now when

I am with my two little boys. In Fallujah, Iraq, they would hit our convoys. We would get a lot of supplies and a lot of the troop movements going in and out of the camp. The insurgents would stand on the bridges over the expressway and shoot the guys as they went by. It doesn't take much to pop up from behind a wall with an RPG and let it fly 30 feet and take out a whole Hummer truck or seven-ton truck. So, I am always leery about people speeding up behind me on the beltway. I am leery, even here in Chicago. I get very leery of overpasses because I always think someone is going to pop up with an RPG and take a shot at us.

I love to run marathons. I couldn't imagine spending my life as a double amputee being 18 years old. It kind of tears you up. They are looking at you trying to talk to you. You have some Marines coming in with their whole leg blown away and they want to go back out and fight insurgents. "Buddy, you are lucky to be alive. You're going home." You get two types. You get the guys who are gung ho and want to go back, and you get the guys who don't want to be there. I think my back ground kind of helped me being there because I was a stronger person. You do a lot of psychiatric care, a lot of talking. Even though we had psych docs there on the combat stress team, you still spend a lot of time doing nursing things like talking to the patients. They are nursing things. They are just different.

I find that I am still having difficulty adjusting. I have been involved in a managed stress work group here at the hospital. There are about six or seven in the group. They are people from Great Lakes Naval Hospital who went over to Iraq. There are a lot of corpsmen. I am the only senior nurse and senior officer in the group. I feel like I have something to contribute to them, and it helps me open up as well. The group is run by one of the social workers.

One of my friends, a colleague, a physician's assistant, was in the same company with me. He works up in the orthopedic clinic. He was having a hard time adjusting when he came back. We talked a lot together. He actually did a short stint over at the VA Hospital as a patient. We don't have a psych service here at this hospital. It was moved to the VA, so folks who need that kind of help go to the VA. The fact that my friend was an inpatient at the VA has kind of disturbed me because it was somebody I know and somebody I served with. I was surprised when he went over there. It made me reexamine my own life.

I had already asked for support. I was one of the first ones when I got back to the command. I went up to mental health and told them that I had issues going on. I couldn't sleep at night. I couldn't lay my head down on the pillow because I always thought they were going to hit us with a mortar or rocket round. I couldn't relax at night. I couldn't watch TV anymore. At night watching the late-night news or watching headline news of combat footage over in Iraq and Baghdad and the green zone and the car bombers would start triggering all this stuff in my head again. I think the medication is helping me relax a little bit. I am also taking Ambien to go to sleep. That has really helped my sleep cycle.

When I came back I didn't feel like I was the same person. I didn't feel like it was my house and my kids. When I left, my son Ryan was 11 months and he was crawling around on my stomach. When I came back he was walking and talking. It was like I missed that whole time period. He didn't even know who I was. When I came home after being gone, it was almost surreal. I went to Iraq into a combat zone and then came back. I woke up one day in my bedroom and looked out the front window at the front lawn. It was just all like a bad dream. I don't feel like it is my own house. I don't feel like the same person. That really bothers me because I don't feel like I am the same husband and father I was. I know it is my house because I bought it. I feel numb everyday when I walk around because of this experience. People tell me things like: "Life could be a lot worse for you." My mother-in-law calls me up from Boston complaining because the garbage man hasn't come for an hour to pick her garbage up and she is all in hysterics. I'm like: "You know, in the big picture of life, it is really not a big deal." For some things I am numb. I don't feel like I am the same person. All my emotions are just gone.

So, when I got back I told them, "I think I need some help. I am not afraid to admit, being a lieutenant and being a nurse, that I'm not right." They asked me when I came back from Camp Pendleton if I had been debriefed. I said "No, no one debriefed us." We didn't talk to any chaplains or anybody. We did our post surveys. My captain in orthopedics, when I worked in the orthopedic clinic here at the hospital, is a very nice man, Captain Paparella. He really cares about his sailors. I sat down with him. He encouraged me to talk and encouraged me to look after the younger guys coming back to say, "Hey, it's okay. It's okay to talk."

That is why I got involved with the combat stress group. The young guys see me as a role model. I don't see that. I just see myself as an active participant in the group with them, sharing the stories that I can share with them. It makes me feel better. It actually gets it off my chest and gets it out. There are a lot of things I can't tell my wife about. There are a lot of things I want to tell her and I can't. I can't talk about it and I am not sure she will understand. I know she understands. It is difficult for me to get it out. I don't know if it is repressed. I don't know if I can ever talk about some issues. I can always talk to the guy I went over with, because we were both there, side by side. He is an orthopedic PA, so he was doing a lot of the surgeries along with me.

Some days I am bothered when I drive down the street and have somebody cutting me off. I sit back in my driver's seat and I'm thinking, "I'm lucky to be alive. If the guy wants to cut me off, let him cut me off." I'm fortunate that I get to drive through the gates of this hospital everyday to come to work.

I am having a hard time coming back here because a lot of people don't even know we have been there. The medical reps come to the hospital and ask, "Have you ever been in Iraq?" "Oh yah, I was deployed for OIF2." "What is OIF2?" "It's the war that is going on in Iraq right now." A lot of people in the United States, in my opinion, have kind of lost focus of what we are doing over there. They have forgotten about it already. In their daily lives all they want to do is complain about the price of gasoline and driving through Dunkin Donuts. I hear a lot of voices, the last time they spoke as they were on the operating room table. I still hear the sounds of people like the medic that I was the one to hear the last words out of his mouth and who died on the operating room table.

I don't have much here in the United States, but I am very appreciative of what I have, like the little material possessions that I own and my two sons, my house, and my '94 Oldsmobile Cutlass that I drive around in. I still like the car. It is little things like that that make me happy and make me appreciate life now a lot more.

My experience in the Gulf changed my work ethic. I always had a strong work ethic, but I do more so now. I just do my job. I hate working with people that are always complaining about something. It is like: "You know, it has got to be done either way." I am trying to pass it along to my corps people. We get these "taskers" now to send people to Kuwait and Afghanistan. Now I have to pick and choose and give names of my corpsmen from the operating room that I am going to send over there. I have a different feeling for it now. It is harder because I am trying to tell them what to expect and what to look out for. Unless you go there and live it, you just won't know.

The whole experience was just so surreal. When I say I woke up in the morning in my bedroom and remembered the dog we operated on and the guy with the bullet in his rib cage, and the Kevlar up in the guy's buttocks, it's like: "Did I really go through all this?" I was there from February 2004 to first of October 2004. It has only been a year since I got home. They tell me it is going to take a while and that is why I am having a hard time adjusting.

I am doing okay at work. Work keeps me busy. It keeps me occupied and doing something productive. I am working on my master's degree, which kind of keeps me focused. When I came back and spoke to the mental health people, they said for me to try and get back into my normal routine as quickly as possible. So, I went right back into the master's program so I could finish it up. It is in management and leadership.

It makes you feel proud and I would go back again. I felt like the whole purpose of everything I ever did in my life from the Coast Guard to being an EMT to being a nurse all came together in this experience. This was what I was supposed to do and why I was here to do it. I was proud to be there and helping the Marines and helping our Army guys and the Iraqi civilians. I even helped with the bad guys. I feel like the Navy trained me to do this and I finally went and did it. It was an experience I will never forget.

I was born in 1960, so when I was growing up we still had people in my neighborhood who were from World War I and World War II. They were older, probably in their 70s or 80s. They would talk about their experiences and I would just sit there in awe. I was just a little kid. I kind of got an understanding of what they actually went through. When I heard them as a little kid, I understood what was important to them, their wives and their children. That was what made life worth living. But they were all very proud to serve. I think about what I will be like in my 70s and 80s as I sit here and people talk about the Gulf War. I am going to react about how proud I feel. I am putting together a little scrapbook for my boys. It is kind of like a living history. That's why I wrote my diary because I don't want to lose all that information. I just wanted to get it down on paper when I got back so I wouldn't lose it. I want to be able to tell my story to my grandchildren someday. Hopefully, they will have some respect for what we did. Hopefully, the Iraqi people will have a good result from what we did.

LAURA FLOOD

Laura graduated from Indiana University with a bachelor's degree in nursing in 1998. After working in the private sector for a period of time, she joined the United States Air Force Nurse Corps in 1999 and landed at Keesler Air Force Medical Center in Biloxi, Mississippi, just in time for 9/11.

I was in mental health when 9/11 happened. I deployed to the Pentagon with a mental health team. That was by far my best experience there. The night of 9/11 everyone got recalled to the hospital. I know the same thing happened at a lot of military bases. We had a rapid deployment medical team and a rapid deployment mental health team. Just by luck or the graces or some political thing, we were the ones that got tasked to go to Fort Dix and wait to see if they needed us. I was originally sent as part of the medical team because I had two specialty codes: one was medical and one was mental health. We got there and they realized they weren't going to need any medical personnel and sent them home. The mental health team advocated keeping me with them because I could be an asset. I was very happy about this. We left from Fort Dix, New Jersey, where we had all been staying and we were bused to the Pentagon. We had a blowout on the way there and stopped at a big truck stop and went in to get something to eat. The truckers saw us all in uniform, and they paid for all of our food and sent us to the front of the line to have our tire fixed. Probably a lot of the truckers were Vietnam vets.

When we got to the Pentagon, it was the middle of the night. We split into day and night shift. We had two social workers, three nurses and five mental health physicians. One doctor was deployed in our big group and then he and one nurse went to a separate facility. They worked in Crystal City and did a lot of family work. We were specifically working with people that were trying to clean up the mess. We split into day and night, and I ended up on night shift for the first two weeks. The last two weeks we were there we all worked together inside the building out of the clinic they had inside the Pentagon. We were called a Critical Incident Stress Debriefing Team.

I enjoyed the night shift the best because we wore badges that said we were part of this team but we really didn't do any large debriefings overnight. We played cards with the guys on their breaks and just let them talk. We did a lot of one-on-one on night shift. We'd sit on the front of the fire truck with the firemen that were on duty and just asked them how they were doing. One of the greatest things was they issued us all cell phones and told us that anybody that needed it could use it free. We let the young guys call their wives and moms.

The Honor Guard was actually the first military guys called up to respond to the Pentagon. Those guys were not prepared. The Honor Guard did a lot of funerals and ceremonies. They were picked because they looked good and all looked about the same. They were completely unprepared to pull dead bodies out of the rubble. Leadership told us that if we found someone that was having a problem and shouldn't be returned to duty that without question they would not be returned to duty. We had a couple of guys we told they couldn't go back. After the first couple of days they sought us out, or they would ask us to come watch TV and then once you got in there and asked how they were doing they would start talking about it. Most of the time they just wanted to say it was awful and know that someone else thought it was awful too.

This effected me more emotionally then any of the flight nursing in Iraq and Afghanistan. The guys coming back from Afghanistan or Iraq hardly ever had complaints about their injuries. They wanted to go back and didn't want to go home. They were positive and energetic and grateful men. What I had to offer them was medical and so it was physical and tangible and everyone knew what to expect. I had some trouble when I came back from the Pentagon, even being a psych nurse, because sometimes you can't identify in yourself what is wrong. When I came back I had a lot of trouble sleeping and I was real jumpy and nervous. Being military you are always concerned that having some mental health problem could impact your career. I asked a social worker I knew if the questions I asked him could be off the record. Of course he threw in: "As long as you're not a threat to yourself or others." I told him I couldn't sleep and I'm jumpy and irritable.

I was walking through the Wal-Mart parking lot late one night, and I had a flash back to this concrete smell and the overhead lights. I couldn't go in. I had to go home. I didn't know why at the time, I just felt instantly nervous and sick. Later I realized it reminded me of all the digging through the rock and concrete and that real sharp smell in the air all the time. They were always in there digging through the stuff and had real bright overhead lights. I only figured that out with my roommate because I said, "Man, I can't understand why I had to get out of there." She said, "Well, you know when you came back you used to tell me that you couldn't get that smell out of your nose." I talked to my social worker friend for a while about it, and he said, "You know what you're describing to me?" I said, "PTSD," and he said, "Well, ya." After it was identified that I was just having some reactions, I was much better.

I had trouble sleeping on and off for almost two years. Slowly it went away. I used to go through two or three nights without getting any sleep and then I'd sleep really hard, and then the next two nights I'd be real restless and then I'd sleep really hard. Now it's just once in a while I have a restless night like that. I can't watch the 9/11 movies that are made. I just don't think it would be a good idea. Some of my patients when I was flying were very gung ho, they would watch that stuff and enjoy it. Others would say they didn't want to have anything to do with it again. I think it was based on their personalities and what kind of jobs they carried in the military.

After the Pentagon I continued working psych for one year. Then I decided it was time to try something else. My chief nurse suggested flight nursing. I had a picture in my mind of it being like ICU. At the time I never had any interest in doing ICU or ER nursing. She had been a flight nurse a couple of times. I told her I wanted something challenging. I was a little irritated that I had been in the Air Force for four years and the war had been kicked off and I had been stuck in Mississippi. At first I said no, and then she told me a little bit more what it was about. I then said maybe. She helped me get the assignments.

I went to six weeks of flight training in Texas. We had survival training on the effects of flight on the neurologic and cardiac cases, pregnancies, etc. We learned what kind of equipment we would have available, since we didn't fly with doctors. It was nurses and technicians in the air. Then I went to Ramstein, Germany, in January of 2005. There is an air medical evacuation squadron there. When I first got there we weren't doing down range missions. We were only flying in the European Theater. Most of Air Force flight nursing is the guard and the reserve. There are only five active duty squadrons. Anymore there are not enough major medical centers overseas that you can fly between. Then they went to universal qualification, where you could fly any patient on any plane. We started flying out of cargo planes. It just slowly switched. I flew from Ramstein to Spain to France and a lot in Italy. It was major injuries that needed to come through definitive care because Ramstein was the major military medical center for all of Europe.

I was able to go a lot of places. We had a deployed unit made up of Navy reserves also at Ramstein, They were the ones going down to Baghdad and Afghanistan and picking these guys up and bringing them back to Germany. We started flying mostly just the ones that went back to the States from Germany. We flew like this for about five months. We'd fly from Ramstein to Walter Reed Medical Center and sometimes we would continue on to San Antonio. A couple of times we flew straight from Germany to San Antonio. It was a very long time in the air.

I was the med crew director and was basically the nurse in charge for the flying medical-surgical unit. We flew with the basic flight nursing crew which was five, two nurses and three techs. They could either augment us up to three nurses and four techs or break us down to one nurse and two techs depending on the requirements. Sometimes we had four or five severely burned patients and would need to go to Texas. When that happened they would just send one nurse and two technicians because we weren't actually doing patient care, we were support for the critical care teams. These teams did the patient care; however, they didn't know anything about the capabilities of the aircraft and how to communicate with the pilot and the patient movement requirement centers around the world. We were there as administration.

Depending on what kind of plane you were on, the C-141 was the one we first started bringing patients back to the States, some of these planes had been in use since Vietnam. I didn't like the C-141s. They called them the tubes of death. They were like a really long skinny tube and it was very dark. They had a pole that went down the middle of the aircraft, and you would hang litter straps from the ceiling. When you brought the litters in, you'd put one side of the litter in the pole in the center and then you'd hang the strap on the other side. You could go up four or five patients high on those. When we had a really full load you could technically take almost 100 litters. Luckily, we usually took between 30 and 40. The C-141s were phased out and replaced with the C-17s. They were bigger and brighter and had these boxes you could bring that had metal arms that went into the floor, and then you could set those litters on these metal arms. There was a lot more space and it was cleaner. They had comfort pallets they could put on there that had flushing toilets and running water. We used a lot of hand gel before that. It had a little cooking area, so we'd make treats and hot dogs and things like that. Some of the Army guys would say they hadn't seen a woman for six months, or they'd smell a chocolate chip cookie and start crying. Every once in a while you'd get one that just hadn't had anything like that. Normally these would be the ones that would be critically injured. We got a lot of burned and orthopedic patients and mental health. I did this for three years.

PATRICIA C. HASEN

Patricia Hasen has seen nursing experience in a multitude of venues. Early in her Navy career she was stationed as a staff nurse at Naval Hospital Oakland and then at the naval hospital in Yokuska, Japan. She worked with the United States Marines at Quantico, Virginia, where she developed an interest in trauma nursing. She was also the facility's VIP nurse, coordinating the visits of many foreign dignitaries and United States military dignitaries both visiting and stationed at Quantico. In 2000 she went to flight school and became a flight nurse, working search and rescue out of Diego Garcia. In 2002 she received orders to Iceland as a special assistant to the outpatient department head. While in Iceland she became the flag aid for the admiral who was in charge of the Iceland Defense Force, Fleet Air Keflavik, and Island Command Iceland. Trish received orders to San Diego Naval Medical Center where she worked in the emergency room

With this wealth of experience, Trish went to Iraq. Her story demonstrates the ability of a nurse to make a difference.

When I was in Diego Garcia I went through 9/11, Operation Enduring Freedom and the bombing of Afghanistan. In Iceland we were building up for Operation Iraqi Freedom. As an aide, I went wherever the admiral went and I had the same security clearance he did. I would go with him into the vaults to do security briefs. We would be receiving information during the briefs. Three times a week we would go into the vault where he would receive followup briefings, and if something came up we would do an on-the-spot debrief. He was part of EUCOM, European Command. EUCOM is all the way through Turkey. EUCOM has been a huge supporter of CENTCOM, or Central Command, which is running the war in Iraq. Because we are part of EUCOM, we also got in on those briefs from EUCOM and CENTCOM. I saw the whole buildup of the war before anybody knew what was going on. It was right there in front of me and I'm a NURSE! I'm thinking, "Oh my goodness gracious." It was fascinating.

It was really, really fascinating what goes on and how you plan a war and what you do to get all these things to happen. Colin Powell, Secretary of State, did a tremendous amount of diplomatic stuff. He would go to nations and talk to them about what our intentions were, what was the benefit to the country, how to get air space. You don't just go to a country and launch Tomahawks across somebody's air space. There was a lot of working in communications on the State Department's side. We had to fly our Tomahawks from the MED (Mediterranean) all the way across to bomb Iraq. It was just fascinating what was going on. I had the opportunity to witness that.

I followed the action of the war. I knew people who were involved in the war. I had one acquaintance, a SWO — surface warfare officer, in Japan. I watched her career. She is now commanding officer (CO) of a ship, the cruiser Winston Churchill. It is the only U.S. ship named after a foreign dignitary. Their navigator was actually a British Royal naval officer. Her ship is in the MED and they carry Tomahawk missiles. We would get reports of what was going on with ships, and I would always watch what was happening with that ship. It is unusual to have a female as CO of a warship. She has had amazing career, and I knew when I knew her in Japan that they were grooming her for FLAG. It was very evident. In Diego Garcia I had a boyfriend who was on a prepositioned ship. They carried bombs and things like that. There were ships that were carrying supplies in and out of the MED. I would watch and make sure, because you know which ships are coming in and out, you would watch for certain ships. My boy friend knew which ships I was looking for, and if he did see them he would say, "That ship looked like the Winston Churchill."

I came to San Diego and I was very blessed. I always said that one job kind of prepares me for the next. It seems divine intervention that it happens. I don't know why I am in such and such a job or what I am supposed to learn from this. But whatever happens, I learn from it and it helps me in my next job.

So, I knew I was coming to San Diego and I sent my senior nurse a letter. I sent my CV and said what I was doing. I hadn't done anything clinical, except take my admiral's blood pressure for a year. I told her to please keep that in mind when she was placing me. I have a lot of ER experience. I have a certification for emergency room nurses and I teach trauma nursing for the Emergency Room Nurses Association. I used to go other places to teach. When I was at Quantico I would go to Defense Medical Readiness Training Institute (DMRI) in San Antonio, Texas. That is where you go to Combat Casualty Care Course. As part of that course, you teach TNCC, Trauma Nursing Core Course. DMRI would fly me from wherever I was to San Antonio where I would teach Friday Night, Saturday night and all day Sunday. You could leave Sunday night, but usually we would leave Monday morning. I worked it out with my boss at OCS that I could do that.

I get the news that I was going to the ER in San Diego. I was concerned about going to this big huge emergency room in this big huge hospital. I was afraid I would flounder. As it turned out, I knew my boss and I also knew the clinical nurse specialist. So, again, I thought it was divine intervention. My department head in San Diego who is now retired, I had met when I was in

Japan. To help me out, my division officer in Japan said, "I can send you to Guam to their ER because of their high acuity. You can get some good experience while you are there in how to triage." I said yes and did a TAD in Guam. I brought a black cloud because they had never cracked open a chest and in the first 30 minutes I was there, the first day, they had to crack a chest. They were sure it was all my fault. It was a fabulous experience. I knew that I could talk to these people and they would help me and they would get me through. I told my division officer, a little teary eyed, "Ma'am, I haven't done clinical for a year. I have been totally outside of medicine." She said, "Trish, it is okay. I know your skills. I know what you did before. You are going to be good." "Well, it is really intimidating going in there." "We will be here. We are not going to have you fail. You are going to do fine." My mentors really help me and I still keep in contact with them, even though some of them are retired now. They were all very helping and certainly not jealous of where I had been or what I had done. I have been very thankful for that.

After I had been in San Diego a month or two in the ER, they said, "We are going to put you on this team and you are going to be in charge of this team." A team in the ER is about eight nurses and eleven or twelve corpsmen. You always work together, so what you put into your team, you get out of your team. You know everybody's strengths and limitations. You build assignments and do things, and you just know how everybody works. You have a vested interest in developing your team because that produces better patient outcomes. So, I was told I would be the team leader and that I would be going to nights pretty soon. Remember, I had been out of clinical for a year. I had just gotten onto this team. There were young lieutenants there who felt they should have been the team leader. They had lots of experience. They had been there a long time. They had a little chip on their shoulders and were a little difficult to work with, but you get through it. I was talking to my department head, and I said, "I hope when they are lieutenant commanders they have lieutenants that are just like them." These lieutenants had deployed. Another deployment was coming up and they were asking for volunteers. Three of the team leaders asked to be deployed. That was interesting because there weren't that many in the whole ER that asked. All the people in my position asked to go. It would have been the second time deploying for one of the people, so she said, "Oh, if somebody else wants to go, that's okay." So, I went in her place. That is how I got to go. I left San Diego on July 17, 2004.

When I was in Iraq I was a flight nurse. I would fly these people that I was amazed that they were still alive. When I would get to the Combat Support Hospital in Baghdad, I would think, "They are alive now, but they are not going to last that long." Then I would see pictures of some of my patients in *Time Magazine* and on the cover of *Newsweek*. Now we have this influx of patients who would have otherwise died because we have advances in surgical capabilities. We have the FRSS/STP (Forward Resuscitative Surgical System/ Shock Trauma Platoon) out there within an hour. We have beefed up the combat casualty care for the medics so they can control hemorrhage with bandages, tourniquets, and quick clot. We are now saving people who would have hemorrhaged out. Because we have Kevlar helmets and body armor, we have a lot of personnel with extremity injuries that would have died previously, but we are saving them. They get to surgery within an hour. We would get fresh trauma injuries or we would get "tail or tail," which means they would come from a forward operating base where they would have had damage control surgery. Then they would come to us to get more surgery. These people are living where they used to die. So now we are seeing brain injuries, spinal cord injuries, traumatic brain injuries that we never saw before because they died. Many people are having TBIs, traumatic brain injury, because a common injury is a blast injury from improvised explosive devices (IED). You may have a blast injury from that, a burn injury, shotgun injuries. So you have a bunch of concomitant injuries. They are finding out that there is a lot of TBI, even just from the blast injury, though they didn't get any shrapnel. Their brain just got knocked around.

You also see TBIs in parajumpers, like the 101st Airborne Division. These guys that are jumping out of aircraft, when they land, they land pretty hard. If you do 200 jumps, you are bound to have some sloshing around of your brain. Now these people are showing up at the MTFs (medical treatment facilities), like Walter Reed, and now to the VA system. We don't really have the capacity to care for all of them, so now there are initiatives in taking care of these people. They find earlier interventions are better. What I want to know is: "What can we do better in the field?"

When I was new to nursing, we documented on paper. There was no data collection. I didn't know about in-route care. All I knew was that I was a flight nurse previously on fixed wing and that easily transposed to rotary wing. So, I teach in-flight care, and we developed a documentation form and we collect data. That is what I want, more of the nerdy: research, wanting information, data back, because that is how we improve our teaching. That is how we understand lessons learned. That is how we improved our programs. That transposes into the clinical side. When you are out there on the flight, you don't have any orders. It's just you, and that can be very hard. You are in total charge of that patient. There are no doctor's orders. You do what is indicated. We, as nurses, are good at doing that because that's what we do as flight nurses, and ICU nurses, too. But if you have multiple patients, they don't do so well because you don't have anything to fall back on if someone questions what you do, unless you have a protocol. Protocols that you work off of right now are basically going to be ACLS protocols, TNCC protocols. We are working on protocols to get those out. I wanted to work on a reference guide, like a pocket guide, that they can use to look things up if they don't know because of our audience and who they are. We are looking at the gear they will have and what improvements we can do to that. That is where my head injury information comes in. We had ICP (intercranial pressure) monitors, but they were not used. The hardest patient to take care of is the head patient, and that is surely complicated if they have an amputation of something and shrapnel wounds and are bleeding. You may have a shock patient who has a head injury, so you aren't going to slam him with fluid for the hypovolemia because they have a head injury. It is like walking a tightrope. You have to balance everything out. That is the hardest piece in the picture. It is that kind of situation that makes me have an interest in that area.

I put on lieutenant commander when I got to San Diego. The admiral put it on via teleconferencing. He was still in Iceland and I was here. I took the oath and my family was here. They put on my boards and I could see the admiral on the TV screen.

We transferred commands to 1st FSSG (Force Service Support Group), 1st Medical Battalion. We went through our exercise in the field. Then you form into what groups you are going to be. I thought they would send me to an STP because I am an ER nurse. But they placed me in Alpha Surgical Company as the senior nurse. I was okay with that. We trained with our group, deployed and we got to Iraq on Friday, the 13th of August. It was a fabulous experience. I always wanted to be deployed. I love the sea. I love the Marines. But you don't know what you don't know. You are on this huge air base. It was Saddam Hussein's air base that we had overtaken.

When I teach flight nursing, I always teach them about the "touchy-feely" said of nursing. There are emotions that you feel that you have never had before. You need to have somebody to talk to when you are having those feelings. In Iraq my roommate was a psychiatrist. Her name was Ann. I think that was divine intervention for both of us. We were a support for each other.

We had dogs on the base. We weren't allowed to have mascots. It was against the rules, but the general before the one that we had, had a mascot dog. There were a bunch of puppies. In our place we had the vet, the one and only vet in that area. He would spay and neuter the dogs and just not say anything about it. He would take care of the dogs for people. We had some medevacs, patients, come through that were suspected to have rabies. We couldn't figure out why we had patients that needed rabies vaccine. We don't even have that vaccine. It was in Baghdad. When you are putting an otherwise healthy patient on a helicopter to go to Baghdad, it was a risk. Every time you fly to Baghdad you fly through what they call "the black zone." It is an area where you have more than a 50 percent chance of being shot at. So there was a big risk involved. We needed to know why these patients had such a risk for getting rabies. It was because they had mascots and there was a mascot that bit two people. The solution was for us to just euthanize all the dogs—knowing Marines were probably antagonizing the dog and the dog bit somebody. I was down in the basement of where I worked and I see the vet with a dog. I said, "Oh, you are spaying another dog? She is beautiful." She is just sitting there in her cage and she has beautiful blue eyes. The vet said, "No, we have to euthanize her." She didn't look sick. I asked what was wrong and he told me what had happened. I was like, "Oh my gosh! Oh yah, in twenty minutes she will be dead."

I got out side and I just started bawling. "What is the matter with me? I am bawling because of this stupid dog. I can't even bawl for my patients, but I'm bawling about this dog." I got back to my room and there was Ann. Thank goodness for Ann. I was just crying and crying. She said, "Trish, what is it? What's wrong with you? What happened?" I told her the story about the dog. "What is wrong with me when I cry for this dog and I can't cry for my patients? What's wrong with me?" "That is the way you cope and that is the way you get on. That's how you can take care of patient after patient after patient." "Okay, I thought something was wrong." It is a coping mechanism.

We did 24-hour duty, meaning the nurses worked 24-hour shifts. There were three of us that worked the floors. Obviously, we didn't stay awake for 24 hours. When it was slow you trained your corpsmen to give IV push antibiotics or hanging the bag if it needed to go into a piggyback. They had the drug and narcotic keys and they get out the narcotics. We count them the next day. I reviewed the notes where they gave them. The patients had good pain control through the night. For an established facility like San Diego, the JCAHO people would be aghast that we gave the corpsmen the narcotic keys and let them push IV antibiotics. But you would never survive in the trauma bays and through a mass casualty if the corpsmen couldn't help you in this way. They better know how to take care of a patient. And they do. We get the patients in on stretchers and put them up on saw horses and they take care of the patients. Granted, they are the most stable patients. But we train them, train them, train them. They are awesome.

My birthday is the 25th of January and I had the duty. That was okay. After all, we were in Iraq. I was resting. One of the people from the HSOC (Health Services Operations Cell), a group that can get on a live chat and kind of get a picture of what is going on in theater, came into the nurses' station where I was sleeping. I was there so the corpsmen could come and get me if they needed anything. The HSOC person came in about three o'clock in the morning and said, "Ma'am, I'm sorry to wake you up. I just need to let you know that a 53 went down." A "53" is a helicopter and a troop transport. I was very concerned because I had friends who were helicopter pilots who were flying that night. I wanted to know where. She said it was out by Korean Village. Then she said the helicopter had been full of Marines. I asked if she had any idea of the status of the people onboard. They didn't have that information, but to standby as we might be getting casualties. So, I got up and made sure I was prepared for casualties. She came back at six o'clock and said we were getting five casualties and may be getting more. These casualties had nothing to do with the helicopter crash. These were fresh casualties from the field. Five casualties is our cut off for taking care of them by ourselves, as the duty crew. After five you have to call mass casualty and everybody comes and then it works really well.

Since it was my duty day, I could choose whatever trauma bay that my team and I would work. As I trained the other nurses, if it was their duty day I would go to them because they were in charge, and say, "Where do you want me? I'm here to help." "Oh, take bay #1. Please take bay #1." Those were the most acute. Of all the nurses, I had the most deaths because those were the most acute patients. When the nurse became more comfortable they would take bay #1 and ask me to take bay #2. You were training your people and you send them on flights with patients that are pretty stable. They probably don't need a nurse to go with them, but you send one for the training. When a critical patient comes through and they volunteer to take the patient, you are very excited for the nurse.

So, on this day patients were coming in and I had bay #1. It was a guy who had massive head wounds. You could see gray and white matter coming out. He had shrapnel injuries. He had tourniquets on. I don't remember whether he lost a limb, but he had these devastating wounds. He still had a pulse and was still kind of breathing. It was pretty amazing. I looked at him and went, "Oh, heck!" because I know I'm going to be flying this guy on because we can't do anything for him there because he had a head injury. He needs a neurosurgeon. I knew I would be flying him to Baghdad. One of the other nurses looks at me and said, "Trish, you know you are going to have to fly him to Baghdad?" "I know, I know." "You know, he may not live." "I'll just hope I can get him there alive. That is the most we can ask for. If we don't go, we won't know." So, I'm getting things ready while they are working on the patient. I needed to follow up on the other nurses. I looked at bay #2 and Rich was on that. I said, "Oh my!" I could see we were going to have to fly this guy, too. He also had a head injury. It wasn't as bad as my guy, but he wasn't doing so well either. Obviously both would get tubed in the trauma bay. I looked around to see what else was going on. I looked at bay #3 and asked Pete, the nurse, how things were going. He said he was doing okay, but that his patient would have to go to the OR. These other guys could go to the OR because they could do something for them, but we would fly the first two out.

I'm thinking about who's going on the trip with me. I have an Army medic and an H-60, which is the helo squadron that I fly with. I knew I couldn't take these two patients by myself because of their devastating injuries. It is our CO who would make the decision, even if a nurse went. He didn't want to lose an asset. If he lost an asset (a nurse, a corpsman), he wasn't getting a replacement. This was the end of our tour, so he was more lenient than he would have been at the beginning or the middle of our tour. There were sometimes when he would not let a nurse go with a patient because he didn't want to lose that asset. If I got shot down or something happened to me, he wasn't going to get a replacement for me. You are constantly weighing resources to risk-benefit. He asked me, "Trish, what do you want; a corpsman or a nurse?" I said, "It doesn't really matter to me, but I need somebody. I can't really do it by myself." "You have your choice. You can take a corpsman or a nurse." So I said, "Rich, do you want to fly?" "Sure, I will go with you. I will fly." So, we got out stuff together and we got the patients out.

The previous trip I had flying, if I thought I was going to die in Iraq, it was that day because the weather was so bad. It wasn't a sand storm. It was like the fog or haze where you can't see in front of your face. It was like when you are in an airplane and you go through a cloud. You look outside and you can't see anything. If you put your hand out, you can't see because it is so thick. That is what it was like.

I was taking a patient to Baghdad or Balad or Abu Ghraib or somewhere. We were coming back. We hit awful, awful weather. We had to fly very low, like 200 or 300 feet off the ground. In a war zone if you are flying higher it is easier to shoot things at you. If you are flying lower, you fly at a faster speed and it is harder to shoot things at you. We were flying at 90 feet because we had to drop down so we could see where we were going. It was just bad. We ended up landing because we couldn't see anything. We were afraid we would run into terrain or we would run into wires or something. I was really saying my prayers that we would make it through. It was not fun. That was the previous flight.

This flight was much better. The weather was clear. That helicopter I talked about before had gone down earlier that night, and we lost 31 people on that flight. We didn't really know why. We had a suspicion it might have been weather, but we didn't know why. At 0700 we are flying and there is not a cloud in the sky. We had clear weather all the way into Baghdad. I had all my equipment and we had a medic with us and I am taking care of these patients. I had a head set on so I could hear, and I told the pilot to tell me when we were ten minutes outside Baghdad. "If you need me to shut up because I am talking to the medic, just tell me." We normally operated that way. When we were ten minutes outside I needed to snow my patients and give them some pain medication because the most turbulent time for patients is take off and landing. I would give the pilot a quick synopsis of what was going on so he could give them report.

I heard the pilot say, "Oh crap!" That's bad. I figured they must have seen something. Then the pilot said, "Ma'am, we aren't getting in there. We aren't going to Baghdad." "Oh, yes we are." "Trish, look out the window." I looked out the window and it was like a curtain of weather. It was like what I had had in my previous flight, which was the worst flight I had ever been on. "Oh shoot, we aren't flying in that. Let's go to Balad." "Balad is closed." So, I am thinking of all the other places that we can go. "What is the closest medical facility that we can get into?' "Al Asad. It is a 45 minute flight." We had just come from Al Asad. That meant that we were going home again.

I have two patients who are intubated. I took oxygen because they were on ventilators. I took oxygen for an hour plus flight. I took sedatives, Versed, for an hour-plus flight for two patients. I had the same with a paralytic vecuronium and fentanyl. It was only enough for one way and then some. I am trying to think what I am going to do. It was bad. I ran out of drugs and oxygen. We had taken them off the vents and we were bagging because we could conserve more that way. It was only five or ten minutes out of Al Asad that we actually ran out of oxygen. But on my guy I couldn't feel a carotid pulse. The medic couldn't feel one either. This was well before the ten minute mark. I can see on the monitor that he is in perfect rhythm, but I can't feel anything, so I have to assume he is in PEA (pulseless electrical activity).

We are doing CPR and I tell the pilot to radio Al Asad and tell them we are coming back. We are not fresh injuries. We aren't somebody else. This is who we are and that we are coming back with those patients. We are doing CPR in route. They were there waiting for us, thankfully. When we got up into the hospital, the staff said we were going to the ICU. I said, "No, these people don't need the ICU. We need to go to the trauma bays." "I was told to take you to the ICU?" "Who told you to take me to the ICU?" "One of the doctors." She knew that there was nothing we could do for these patients, so they would become "expectant." My guy did have a pulse and we were bagging him. I just couldn't feel it in the aircraft because he was so hypovolemic. We got them to ICU and put them on the vents. The doctor came in and said, "Take them off the vent." I looked at her and she said, "Take him off the vent." So, I took him off the vent. She was listening and I was feeling for a pulse. She said to put him back on the vent. I was grateful because I didn't want to kill my patient that way. There was nothing we could do for this patient. We just waited until he died. It took about ten minutes.

I could hear the family practitioner doc who was behind me freaking out about the second patient. I could hear the nurse tell the doctor, "The blood pressure is 60/20." I could hear the other doc saying, "Get the ACLS drugs." I looked at my doctor and said, "He wants to resuscitate. Tell him to stop." She finally got his attention and said, "Stop. Just let him go. You aren't going to save him. He's going to die. Just let him go." She had to repeat it several times. They let him go. He died about five minutes after the first patient.

I had a hard time with that. It was my birthday. We had just lost 31 people on the helo. Then this flight. It was very hard. I had a hard time dealing with that because I had never experienced those feelings. I never lost a patient in flight, never in Diego Garcia or in Iraq. I felt like they were in my total charge, and I felt like I let them down. So, when I am teaching I tell my students to learn from my experiences. I tell them to take plenty of oxygen. You take plenty of drugs. You plan for a contingency if you can't get in one place and you have to go someplace else or you have to land in the middle of nowhere because you can't see where you are going. You plan. Learn from my mistakes. Let me tell you how the feeling part goes. I plant those seeds that it is okay to talk about it. It is okay to say, "This is what I am feeling and I have never felt this way before."

I talked with someone who said, "I walked into the OR and there was a hand in a bucket because they had done an amputation and I thought, 'Oh, it's a hand.'" He just went on and got report. He said, "Trish, I had no emotion. What is the matter with me?" I went back and I said, "That is how you cope. You'll never forget it. It will never leave you, but that is how you cope. One day you will have to deal with that."

You have this patient who is totally, 100 percent in your charge. I have been in trauma bays and in ERs and you work as a team and the doctor is the team leader. You do all you can do and everybody has input into it. You ask if anybody has any other ideas. And you call the code. But it was always a team effort. There was always that doctor there in charge. But in situations like our flight, you are 100 percent in charge. I had never felt like that before, and I had never lost a patient in flight before. It is really, really hard. I talked to the Catholic father about it because it really shook me up. "Father, I am really having a hard time with this. Why did it have to happen? It was crystal clear blue skies. My patients would have made it there alive. I would have gotten them there alive. I don't know what would have happened after that. I don't know if they would have gotten to see their family or their family would have gotten to see them. We came back and they were technically alive when we landed, but I can't get over that I lost them." He said, "Whatever the reason was, those boys were going to die. Just look at all the things that happened that day. For whatever reason, you were supposed to learn something from this."

I learned a lot. You look at the quality of life these people had and what they have now, look at how they would live their lives. These are healthy, robust young men. One was 19 and the other was 21. They would have to deal with these injuries for the rest of their lives. For some reason they weren't supposed to live. Whatever the reason was, it didn't happen for them to live. Whatever lessons were learned or whatever the outcomes were supposed to be, they were not supposed to make it. It is just interesting how God has his hand in everything.

JERRY R. HILL

Jerry Hill graduated from North Michigan University with a bachelor's degree in nursing 1971. He enjoyed high-pressure, high-stress, challenging work and so decided to return to receive his degree as a nurse anesthetist from Hurley Medical Center in Flint, Michigan, in 1979. He found working as a nurse anesthetist in smaller communities provided the satisfaction of an independent nursing practice. Jerry's ability to practice independently, to set priorities and make required decisions allowed him to make a difference in the lives of his heroes.

I love history, especially World War II. I've read a lot of books on World War II about the soldiers and the Marines, and it was incredible being gone for three and four years, not knowing if you'd come back with the high casualty rates. Those guys became my heroes. The heroes are the guys that go out and put their lives on the line for our country. By George, they did their duty and they did their jobs and they really became my heroes.

I began to develop a deep sense of patriotism and wanted to be a part of that military community and culture. I was in college at the height of the Vietnam War. I was in college, married, and having a family, so military life was not an option for me at that time, but I always wanted to be part of that group. After my kids got a little bit older and family was a little bit more stable, I began to look into the reserves. I'd had two years of ROTC in the Air Force, so I first looked into the Air Force Reserve. I was 39 years old, and they told me I was too old.

My kids were playing hockey at the time. I happened to run into another hockey dad. I told him, "I always wanted to join the reserves, and I actually had always wanted to join the Navy, but in the upper peninsula of Michigan in the Midwest there's not a whole lot there." And he said, "Why don't you join the Navy reserve. There's one five miles from your house." I checked that out immediately and found out that there was a Navy reserve facility within ten miles of where I lived. It just so happened at that the Navy had raised the age limit to 45. From the time that I found out there was a Navy reserve facility, it was 60 days until I had my commission.

I started doing a weekend a month, and my family was supportive. I knew there was a possibility of going to war. They knew that deep down inside, it's what I wanted. The reason I joined the Navy was to be in the middle of the alligators, in the middle of combat, saving the lives of my heroes. Iraq invaded Kuwait in 1991, and I thought, "Here's my chance. Here I go!" I had been in the Navy at that time for two years. I got my boots out of the closet and started wearing them all day around the house, getting them broke in. We were going to be called. I knew it. We were going to do it. I kept waiting for the word. Everybody would say, "You called up yet?" "Nope, nothing." Never heard, never heard, never heard, and then all of a sudden the war was over, and I never got called out. I would see these guys coming home, the parades, and all that stuff, and I thought, "I wanted to be a part of that club." I love my two week ATs. They are great, but they didn't make up for the actual action of being mobilized. I've been to Italy, Iceland, Camp Pendleton, Twenty-nine Palms, and Jacksonville several times. I tried to get my training at every platform that the Navy had, whether it was a camp hospital out in the desert or out on a ship or on a brick-and-mortar thing, so if I ever did get called out, I would know a little bit about the environment. I was discouraged when I didn't get called out. Of course my family was happy that I didn't, but I was discouraged.

    I went back to the training. It was a big joke in the Navy at that time. I'd

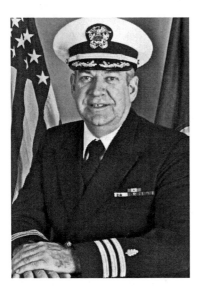

This picture was taken August 2004, just prior to Commander Hill's deployment to Iraq. Commander Hill currently practices as a nurse anesthetist at Baraga County Memorial Hospital in L'Anse, Michigan.

only been in at that time a few years, but now I have been in a total of 16 years. I've only been on the ship once. The rest of the time was spent in the desert. You don't even see water, but we support the Marines, so we go where the Marines go.

    I continued doing my two week job. In 2003 President Bush decided to finish what his dad didn't finish, so we went to war with Iraq. In two months or less the war would be over, or so we thought. Then it was kind of funny. I'd had a lecture in the reserve center about how they choose people for active duty. Supposedly at that time I was told they would go through the list and see if they needed, let's say, a nurse anesthetist. They would see how many ensigns were available, and take them first, and then they would take JGs, then the lieutenants, and lieutenant commanders, and then the commanders. I'm a commander, and I have five years experience as a commander. I don't think I'm going to be called. It's not going to happen. I was so discouraged. I thought I was going to spend 20 years in the reserve and never go on active duty. I realize that I did my part and nobody is going to criticize that, but there's not going to be that satisfaction. That's not what I joined for. June 2004, on a Thursday afternoon, I get this call from the reserve center saying, "We got some news for you. Are you sitting down?" And I thought, "Oh, I'm getting promoted to captain." And they said, "You're being mobilized. You're being recalled." In the early part of 2003, I had gone so far as to make some phone calls to see if I could volunteer for active duty and get sent over to Iraq. I was told, "Yeah, you can volunteer for active duty, but where you're going to go will be up to the Navy. We cannot guarantee you'll be sent overseas." I thought, "If I go, I want to be in combat, with the people. I don't want to be sent somewhere else in a brick-and-mortar place, because for one thing, I'm going to take a horrible financial hit." The military pay is less than half of my civilian pay and with no guarantees. I said I'd just sit tight.

That Thursday night I got a call and they said, "You're being recalled. We don't know when. We don't know where you're going to go. We don't have your orders yet. They're supposed to come in tomorrow; and as soon as they do, we'll give you a call and let you know." I got the call the next morning saying, "You have a one year recall. You're to report to the reserve center Monday morning. You're being assigned to Naval Hospital Camp Pendleton." So they gave me one weekend.

By this time I'd been divorced. I lived by myself. I had a business on the side, and all of a sudden I had two days to close my house off, pay my bills, take care of my dogs, and all of that stuff, to be gone for a whole year's time. Fortunately, I had paid attention to the people in the reserve that said, "Always have your affairs in order because you could be called at any time." I followed that. I had a list of all of my creditors and phone numbers. I was able, over that weekend, to pack up, get my financial situation taken care of, close my house off, have people take care of my dogs. Fortunately, my daughter and son-in-law lived 15 miles away, so they could keep an eye on it, keep the snow plowed in the wintertime so the fuel truck could get in and keep the furnace going, and that sort of thing.

I reported for duty. I was sent out to Camp Pendleton Naval Hospital. I was being processed in at Great Lakes, but called the reserve liaison officer at Camp Pendleton and said, "What's the chance of me going to Iraq?" They said "Zero. You're going to be backfill for Naval Hospital Camp Pendleton, and you won't have to go overseas." I said, "But I want to go overseas. If I'm going to be recalled for a year, I want to go over to Iraq. Is there any way I can do that?" He said, "Well, it's possible. Let me make some phone calls and see what happens." A week later when I reported for duty and I reported to him, I said, "Is there any possibility of us going to Iraq?" He said, "Well, they need four anesthesia providers over there. They are asking for four anesthesiologists.

I will send an e-mail and see if we can substitute one or more of those anes-
thesiology billets for a nurse anesthetist instead." He got an e-mail back and
they said they would be willing to substitute ONE of those slots for a nurse
anesthetist, but the rest had to be anesthesiologists. I said, "Can I have it? I
want it. Sign me up for that slot!" He said, "Are you sure that's what you want
to do?" I said, "That's what I want to do." He said, "Okay." My department
head of anesthesia at Camp Pendleton had been the fourth anesthesiologist
slated to go, so of course it broke her heart. I was going to go in her place.
She's a nice gal. I like her.

The bricks fell into place, and I was able to go to Iraq. I went with the
first medical battalion out of Camp Pendleton. There were a 138 medical people
to be spread out to Iraq. I was the only reservist in that group. I was 55 —
much more "mature" than the others. I knew coming from a cold weather cli-
mate that I wasn't going to like the heat, and that was going to be hard. I also
knew that I would have to pull my weight. I couldn't slow any one down. If
that meant to hump a mile with a pack on my back, I was going to do it to
keep up with the rest of the kids. I got my mind straight that I was not going
to be any type of a slacker or burden.

My whole focus was on the mission, what we were going to do. I didn't
care about the living condition. I didn't care what happened to me. If I died
over there, that was okay with me. I made my peace with everybody before I
left. My business affairs were all tied up before I left. I said my final good-
byes to everyone. I actually left to Iraq with a completely clean slate. Anything
that needed to be said to anybody, any forgiveness that needed to be forgiven,
any affairs all the way around the line, that was all done and taken care of. In
a way it was kind of like my whole life came together. I had everything taken
care of while I was gone. I'm not one that's going to paint a target on my chest
and run out there. But at the same time, I wasn't afraid of whatever fate awaited
me. I was willing to accept that fate. I was going to be with my heroes and my
guys, and I was going to do the best job that I could do.

We bussed from Pendleton to March Air Force Base. From March we
flew into Kuwait City. We got into Kuwait City at one or two in the morning.
It was a 115 degrees at that time. I thought, "Here it goes. Just suck it up guy,
suck it up." I think back in World War II and in Vietnam, these guys were in
the jungle in 100 degree heat, day after day and exposed to the elements. In
Europe it was snow up to their eyeballs and that kind of stuff. They had it a
lot worse than what I was going to have. There's not going to be any complaining here. I'm just going to suck it up. It was hot. We flew out the next
day from Kuwait City to Iraq. We flew in on a C-130. That was probably the
most physically, stressful day that I had in my entire experience. When we left
Kuwait City it was two in the afternoon. It was over 130 degrees that day. It
was just so dawg-awful hot.

The heat is just debilitating. It was just so hot. They put us in the back of a C-130 — two rows of seats facing each other on each side of the plane, so there were four rows of seats. They pushed us so tight in there that our shoulders were literally tight against the person sitting in the middle of you. The person sitting across from you was so close you had to alternate your knees, and your knees were about two inches from the other person's crotch. That's how close we were. Then they start passing the equipment down, duffel bags and backpacks and camel backs. Everything was piled up on your lap almost to your chin. This is in 135 degree heat in a C-130, and then they close the rear door, and we sat in that runway for an hour before we took off. Temperatures inside that plane had to be between 165–175 degrees. It was just awful, absolutely awful! Then we flew to Iraq. They never flew any higher than 300 feet. I don't know why they fly close to the ground. I've never been able to figure that out. I'm sure there's a reason, less radar maybe. I would think your short-range missiles would worry you more. We flew for about two hours, no windows open. It was just stuffy. We had our camel backs on, drinking the fluids, but those camel backs were almost empty by the time that we took off. Besides that, you were packed in there so tight you couldn't move an ankle or a leg. You couldn't adjust your position. You couldn't stand up or move. It was torture, really bad. About 20 minutes out from that flight, I just started vomiting like crazy. Fortunately, I had a plastic bag in my pack so I didn't have to vomit down my shirt or in my helmet, which some of the others had to do. I was probably on the verge of heatstroke by the time we landed. I was sick for two days. I couldn't eat. I was so dehydrated, just incredibly, incredibly ill. There were other people, but I was probably the worst. The younger ones tolerated it better, but I like cold weather. It was a combination of fluids and air sick. The combination of being cramped tight in the heat, not having the fluids, being that close to the ground and having it bumpy all contributed to me being ill. I wasn't in bed, I could get up and walk around, but I had no appetite. I just felt nauseated. They put us in Al Asad, which is an air base, or a big Marine base in Iraq. That's where they fly everybody. It's the central processing plant. Everybody that flies into Iraq flies into Al Asad. They put us in C-huts. We were there for seven to ten days before we were transferred to our final destination.

In Al Asad our chow hall was probably about a mile from where we were berthed, and you really had to want to eat. It was easier to get an MRE than go to the chow hall. The chow hall was excellent there. The food there was really good, no problem with that. Lots of times we would walk down in the morning when it was cool, and late at night for dinner. It was not open 24 hours. They had specific hours for breakfast, for lunch maybe 11–1 and dinner was like 5–7 or something. But the food there was excellent.

When we got off that plane and flew into Al Asad, they said, "There's no water, so there'll be no showers for at least seven days." They had brought some bottled water for us. They had the shower stalls there. So I would take three bottles of water with me and stand in the shower and pour one bottle over me: I would soap up with that and then use two bottles of water to rinse off. It was really common. Not that big of deal. At least we had some place to take a shower and have a little bit of water. Again, I'm thinking back to World War II. They had none of that stuff.

We had no place to do our laundry. I had about ten or twelve T-shirts that I had brought with me, and that's the part that would really get soaked. We would wear our uniforms for about four days and then switch to others, so by the time we were ready to get to our final destination, I still had enough clothes. Before I left I took a pair of underwear, a pair of socks, and a T-shirt and put them in a plastic bag and sealed it off. So each day I just had to reach into my duffel bag, pull out a plastic bag, and I had clean stuff for that day. I wore the same uniform over and over until it got so bad I would just stuff that away. I had three sets of uniforms with me, so I didn't have to do any laundry.

Because there is no running water for our toilet facilities, we just had port-a-johns. You can imagine what 30 port-a-johns are like in a 130 degree heat. Your time in the port-a-john was as long as you could hold your breath and that was just about it. In fact, it was so bad there, that you had to have what we called a combat buddy. Whenever you had to use the port-a-john, you had to bring a buddy with you that would stand outside, because it was so hot in those port-a-johns they would have people pass out. Obviously, if somebody passed out in there and no one knew they were in there, they would die of heatstroke. You would have people standing out there saying, "Are you okay in there?" "Yeah, everything's fine." But if it got silent and they didn't answer back, they'd tear that door right off. It was really a shock. It wasn't just the sudden environmental change. You had to have a combat buddy with you to go in the bathroom.

I think of security. They were worried about insurgents kidnapping people. There were still Iraqis on base. You'd assume they were the good guys, but you didn't know for sure, so you didn't want anybody being alone by themselves and getting kidnapped and ending up on Al Jazeera or on TV. It was kind of joke amongst us. "You're going to go by yourself? We'll wave at you when we see you on TV." There's a reason for that. They just didn't want people to be alone. They wanted people to look out for each other and make sure everybody was okay.

Accountability of personnel was an issue. They wanted to make sure everybody was there, because that is a huge base out there in Al Asad. You go wandering off there and get lost someplace, you might never get back. You could easily die of heatstroke or heat exhaustion if you got out in that desert in that heat and got lost. They want to make sure that everybody's around. The commanding officers did a good job of telling everybody to keep track of so and so. We had roll call two or three times a day to make sure everybody was there and accounted for. If somebody was missing (and that did happen several times), we went through every barrack and everything until that person was found. They weren't lost; they had just decided to go to the internet café or the chow hall on their own. There was one guy that seemed to be our perennial lostee. He was a young Marine that just didn't seem like he had his act together at all. We would find his ID lying out in the desert on the ground some place, his mind was somewhere else all the time. He was a nice kid. He wasn't a trouble maker or bad. He was just kind of a goofus. His mind was just in a different world than most of ours. He was always losing stuff. He'd be the one missing and we'd go find him. He'd be sleeping back in some tent in the corner someplace, or he decided he'd go get something to eat, just never stayed with the group.

We were in Al Asad about 7–10 days, and from there I was assigned to a Marine base called Korean Village, which was about 30 miles from the Jordanian border in western Iraq. We just waited for transportation. Al Asad, the big transportation hub, had so many helicopters transporting people — hundreds and hundreds of Marines coming into the base every day — so we just had to wait to get our name on the flight manifest. There were several times we got all of our gear packed up, got on the palate, on the bus, and then they would say, "There's been a change the schedule. A priority has come up. You're not going out tonight." And then you would haul all your stuff back to your room and wait maybe till the next day, or maybe the next hour and then you were going to go at two o' clock, and then it was six o'clock, and then it was midnight. Finally, about midnight, we got the opportunity to go to our final place.

Some of our group were assigned to the hospital in Al Asad. There were 138 of us. We were broken up into groups, some at Fallujah, some at Al Taqqadum, some at Al Asad, some at Madiasis, some at Korean Village, some at Al-kan. That was pretty much the group everybody was distributed to. I was assigned to an FRSS, a forward resuscitating surgical system at Korean Village. There was also an STP, so there were 28 of us that were assigned at Korean Village. Basically, what Korean Village is and the reason it got that name is because it's located right beside a four-lane highway that comes out of Syria and Jordan, hooks together, and goes into Baghdad. I'm assuming the highway was built back in the '50s or '60s. They had built this little city for Korean contractors, and that was their housing there. It was totally abandoned — no windows, no doors, just cement buildings surrounded by a six-foot wall all the way around it. They had doors and windows when they lived there, but they had nothing there for the past 10 or 15 years. When the Army took over in 2003, they put in windows and doors and kind of rehabilitated it, put a little electricity and generators and wiring and that sort of thing, but there was no indoor plumbing per se or anything like that whatsoever. It was a very remote outpost; it was more like a staging area.

We had 1,000 Marines assigned to that base. That was their staging area. They would send groups of 50 and 100 to the Jordanian border, the Syrian border, and Saudi Arabian border to do border control. Iraq borders Syria, Jordan, Saudi Arabia, Iran, and Kuwait. Our area of responsibility was the border from Syria to about halfway up because Al-kan was about halfway up. They also had a responsibility for that border. The entire Jordanian border was our responsibility and about 280 miles of the Saudi Arabia border. Basically our unit was an STP and an SRS unit on this little tiny base. The Marines would go out to the border areas, and then if there were any incidents or injuries or whatever, we had an Army medic and two Black Hawk helicopters at that base. They would medevac the people, bring them back to us and then we would treat them. We got a lot of emergency-type patients, but our surgical unit was hardly used at all. The people before us, in the 18 months that the military had provided that base, had had one surgery that took place. It wasn't even a necessary surgery; it was kind of one they could do while they were waiting for the helicopter. It wasn't even required.

At that point I realized that was why they had allowed one nurse anesthetist instead of the anesthesiologist because they knew they were going to stick me out in this base where they knew I wasn't going to be used. That was discouraging. I knew that was kind of the thinking that went on there. Most units had two surgeons to it. We had one there because they knew they weren't going to be used. They needed a body; they needed to be able to tell the Marines, "We have this operating room set up there if you get hurt," but knowing the chances of that were very small. It's possible we could've been needed, but based on the history of the place, they knew if it was used it was going to be very minimal. I never saw anybody in surgery the whole time I was there. I helped in the emergency room. I don't know what our total count was, but we were there for six months and we saw probably 200. Some were pretty severe injuries, some gunshot wounds to the chest, some Iraqis with that. We got some IEDs with some partial amputation of some legs, a lot of shrapnel injuries, a lot of vehicle rollovers. We saw a fair number. I was able to be used to help start IVs and intubate patients, just kind of help out. But if it hadn't of been for Fallujah, I would have been very disappointed.

Early in September of 2004 we got word that we would be planning a major operation in Fallujah. We were going to take that city down. We were going to clean the rat's nest out of there. They knew it would probably be the biggest battle since Vietnam. This was going to be about 10,000 Marines against minimum 3,000 insurgents, who are very well embedded. We knew we would fight to the death, and we knew we would probably get a whole lot of casualties for it. To the military's credit, Fallujah had three operating rooms, but they only had one anesthesiologist and one nurse anesthetist. They could only use two operating rooms. They thought they should keep open that third operating room, at least during the time Fallujah was going on. There weren't any other anesthesia providers throughout Iraq that they felt they could pull out and use, because the ones in the other areas were fairly busy. They were doing surgeries in those other FRSSs. We were the only ones that weren't doing anything at all. They felt they could roll the dice and pull me out of Korean Village and put me there for three weeks to a month, maybe six weeks. They told me I would be there about a month. They would not have any surgical services available at Korean Village because there would not be an anesthesia provider. They felt the chances of my being used at Fallujah were a whole lot more than me being used at Korean Village.

At the time they told me I would probably set up there I thought, "This is great!" Every time they came around and said there was a possibility, I was saying, "Hey, I volunteer. If you need me, I'm willing to go. Do you want me to go tomorrow? I have no problems with this." The surgeon would have liked to have gone, too, but they said they had enough surgeons up there. The surgeon was going to sit there with our whole surgical team in Korean Village. We tried to say, "Why don't you bring our whole surgery team up. Number one, you can never have enough help in a nasty combat situation. Number two, morale wise, it will give our team a sense of accomplishment. Number three, it will be excellent training for the people. We're not doing any cases up here month after month. It'll help keep their skills up." But the decision was made that we would have to convoy up there, and our convoys were getting hit with IEDs a lot. They felt like they had enough people with the exception of another anesthesia provider, and they would be putting them at risk of death or injury during the transportation to get there. That was the reason they didn't take up our whole team. They were very disappointed. They really wanted to come too.

All of us are in the military and in the medical field to take care of people. We don't want to be sitting around all day doing nothing. All of us felt we were set out there to rot, the surgical team anyway. We even told the commanding generals when they came around to visit us and they were making plans as to what medical personnel they needed. We were telling them, "Don't send a surgical team out here. Don't pull someone from home to send them here if they are not needed. Keep the emergency room, but you don't need a surgical team here." We tried to tell them not to send a team. They didn't listen. The way it turned out was when we got ready to leave, there was no surgical team there; but at the very last minute one of the Marine commanding generals saw we had no surgical team available, and he said, "No surgical team available? We must have surgical capabilities for every Marine within one hour of whatever Marine deployed. That is our doctrine. That is our policy, and if they sit out there and rot for six months, that's great, because no Marines got hurt." It's hard to argue with that, and they were scrambling to pull a surgical team in there. Some people got a last minute notice that they were going to Iraq that didn't expect to go. As we were at Al Asad on the way home, we saw the surgical team that would be heading down.

What they decided to do in Fallujah was pull me up there to work at the hospital and open up a third operating room. They would also open up another STP at the edge of the city. They pulled our one doctor and nurse that were down at Mediasis up, they pulled one of our physician assistants and two or three of our corpsmen up, and they augmented them with one or two corpsmen from Al Taqqadum to form an eight or nine person STP at Fallujah. We were all helicoptered up to Fallujah together.

They told us to expect 200 casualties within what they thought would be a three weeks' battle. At the end of the first week, we had treated 411 patients in the emergency room, and out of those we had treated 200 surgical patients. In the whole operation I think we treated 500 or so people. It took about seven days to take that city down. They moved much quicker than they had thought. I wanted to be up to my butt in alligators and we were. Before Fallujah, we were getting 10–15 patients a day, some days only five or six patients a day. We were doing over 70 a day when Fallujah hit. After that first week it was 20 and 15, and by the time I left it was back to almost nothing. The big push was the first seven to ten days. We were literally doing all we could handle. Fortunately, the Marines did a good job of staggering who was going to get shot, because we would no sooner finish up then we would get a call, "We're getting eight more urgent surgicals coming in." We could divide up those eight into the more critical, and we would get those eight taken care of; and then as soon as we were finishing up our last, we would get a call, "Ten more urgent surgicals coming up." They came in continuously. Because we kept that third operating room open, there was never a severely injured Marine waiting to go into surgery. We were able to keep up. Anybody that needed surgery, we were able to get to them right away.

We did meatball surgery there. We would wash out wounds, stop the bleeding. We did a lot of vein graft surgery, arteries that were severed that we had to use vein grafts and put them back together. We got a lot of arm, brachial arteries severed. We got a lot of those, but nobody died waiting for surgery. We were able to get them, and then we would fly them out. Some days we were sending 30 to 40 surgical patients to Baghdad. We sent any surgical patients to Baghdad and Balad. Any insurgents that were treated were sent to the Army hospital at Abu Ghraib. We treated insurgents, civilians, the Iraqi National Guard that was fighting with us, and Marines and soldiers.

I remember one patient that will always, always be with me. He was a young Army guy. When he first came in we took the bandages off his belly and we thought we saw this live mortar round in his belly. We saw this metal fin sticking out in his belly, and we thought, "What are we going to do. Everybody clear out. He's got a live mortar in his guts!" But the Army medic who had brought him in said no. She had taken him to the EOD (Explosive Ordinance Division) before she brought him. They had checked it, but this was not live; this was a detonated one. She was smart. She did an excellent job. She was an Army medic, and she was out there with those guys. I'd seen her bring in several guys in those weeks, and she was good. Those Army medics were excellent. We pulled the bandages off and he had suffered a complete evisceration. His intestines and his bladder were gone. Everything between two inches above the belly button to the pelvic bone was gone. And he was still alive. The ER docs said, "He's had a complete evisceration. We've never ever had anyone survive a complete evisceration. There's no sense in wasting surgical assets on this guy. He's not going to live." At that point the Army medic that had carried him broke down and just started crying. She had tried so hard to save this man's life. Our doctor kind of felt bad for her, and he said, "Well, we'll see what we can do." So they did an ER thoracotomy. They opened up his chest to see if he had any heart beat or anything going in his heart, and his heart was beating. He wasn't responding, but we checked his pupils and his pupils were equal and dilating, this kid wasn't dead. He was still alive. In deference to her, they brought him in the OR and I was his anesthesia provider.

We opened him up and explored, and found that our initial diagnosis was correct. His injuries were not life sustaining. Everything was gone — not only his intestines, bladder, but everything was gone. The doctor felt that the abdominal cavity had fecal contamination, that even if they got him off the table alive, he would die within two or three days. There's no way he's going to survive his injuries. There was nothing that could be done. We were just going to pack his abdomen, stop the blood, stop the fluids, and just let him go. Of course, we have him on a heart monitor, still have him on the ventilator, and we've given him medication to paralyze him, so I can't take him off the ventilator and basically suffocate him. The doctors said, "We're just going to let him go." So I stayed with that kid for an hour and a half before he died, just standing there. He didn't wake up at all, but sometimes surgery wise, they can still hear. You don't know. Obviously he's in deep shock, and we don't know if he still might possibly hear. We stayed with him and we talked to him. In a way we told him what was happening. We told him we were proud of him, that he was a good soldier, and that it was okay to go. We told him he would be in a better place. We had the priest with him, who talked to him and prayed with him. It was like having a funeral service for someone that was still alive. Tough stuff. About an hour and a half later his heart gave up and he died. It's not only seeing some 19-year-old die like that, it's just the helpless-ness; but that's what we were there to do. We knew that we're going to see patients like that. So you do the best you can at that time. It's harder now to talk about it than it was at the time.

Once we took the patient into the operating room, the Army medic prob-ably left and went back to her unit to provide other help. I'm sure she got word next time she came to the hospital that he didn't make it. She knew he wasn't going to make it. She had done everything *she* could do for him. She wanted us to do everything *we* could do for him. And we did. There's no regret on my part. Could we have done something else? We did all that we could do. It's just the helplessness of not being able to help that kid.

We had another kid that kicked down a door, and insurgents threw a grenade at his feet and blew both of his legs off. He had some intestinal injuries and some arm injuries. We worked on him for a long time. We gave him about 17 units of blood. I have a picture of the hallway of the hospital at Fallujah with the operating room door closed. Blood was running underneath the oper-ating room door into the hallway. The blood was literally flowing from the operating room into the hallway on some of the injuries. Of course we're pumping massive amounts of blood into these patients. The only thing I think our doctors were going to recommend and the biggest thing we could've done better was that we had no clotting agents. We knew we would be getting some serious wounds, but we had no fresh frozen plasma, no clotting agents. This kid who we'd given 17 units of blood was beginning to bleed out. We activated the walking blood bank and gave him some fresh blood to hope for the clotting agents. We did get him off the operating room table, but he was in severe shock and on vasopressors. He died on the helicopter on the way to Baghdad. We just couldn't stop the bleeding on him. He just bled and bled and bled. That would be "lessons learned." There's a lot to do to set up a unit like that, but when you know you're going to be getting a lot of casualties for a month, that investment should be seriously looked at. If you're going to be going to all this work to save people, you should be willing to do that. Most of the rest of the injuries were a lot of extremity injuries because our Marines are wearing the flack and Kevlar units.

We had to fill out a report on every patient that we got over there. I think it was four pages all together, questions like: "Were they wearing their flack and kevlar at the time? Where were the injuries located? Did the flack and kevlar help?" They were putting it in a big study. They had two or three guys that all they would do is fly from place to place collecting these forms and showing people how to fill these forms out. These forms were going back to the manufacturers of the body armor company to see where the weaknesses were in the body armor, to see where the different injuries were being located. They wanted to improve and redesign the armor in the future, but there is only so much armor you can put on and still be mobile. As a result, a lot of guys hit by RPGs and mortar wounds would come in with their arms and legs lacerated to pieces. They were alive, because their body armor had protected them, whereas in other wars they would have been killed. The fragments would have gone through their chest also.

We would have cases where I was working with two general surgeons and two orthopedic surgeons for one patient. A lot of extremity injuries. It was an orthopedic surgeon's either worst nightmare or paradise, depending on how much carpenter work you wanted to do. They had pulled an extra orthopedic surgeon to work out there during that time.

That was the high point of my Navy career. As nasty as it was, I wrote a letter home saying, "I am surrounded by death, misery, and destruction, and pure hell, and I love every minute of it." That's what I'm there for, what 16 years of reserve training were put in for. I got to do what I'd always hoped to be able to do. I had that satisfaction of doing being part of that team.

Another thing that happened during Fallujah besides just getting patient after patient, we were literally getting two hours of sleep a day for those seven days. We were beyond exhausted. You were just living on pure adrenaline. We had a little bit of a break in the action when we had about 30 minutes to an hour, and the anesthesiologist there told me, "Go to the chow hall and get something to eat." We were living on Oreos and M&M's and crackers and care packages people had sent. The chow hall was a half a mile away or more away, and we didn't want to take the time to go out and eat. Besides, we were too darn tired to walk down. They would bring us something now and then every two or three days. It was just grabbing what we could get, because we were too tired to do anything else. I remember having a little bit of time off, and all I wanted to do was go have a shower, and stand under that shower and reenergize and refresh myself. That's all I wanted to do. I went to the shower and it was a real shower, which was nice. We didn't have real showers at Korean Village. We had shower tents. They had real showers where you could stand under the shower for as long as you wanted. I remember standing under that hot water for 10–15 minutes decompressing, reenergizing, and going back.

There was an artillery battery at Fallujah. It seemed like they were in the hallway of the hospital. I honestly don't know how close they were, but they were close enough that every time an artillery round would go off, the building would shake and dust would come up off the floor. Those first seven days, it NEVER stopped. It was going off every 10 to 15 seconds, and the windows would just rattle, even if you were able to go lay down, it was like being inside a clothes dryer. The constant noise never stopped. Psychologically, I just wanted to go to the artillery battery and yell, "Will you guys just stop it! Stop it! Just give me 15 minutes and just stop it!" I thought, as bad as I have got it here, listening to these rounds going off constantly, what must it be like to be on the receiving end of these shells. That must have been just awful, because psychologically it stressed me out. I imagined it could push people over the edge. In the first 24 hours they fired more artillery rounds than they had the entire year before that. That artillery battery just never quit. Finally after the first week when it had settled down, there would be little hotbeds, and all of a sudden the artillery battery would let loose. At two, three, four o'clock in the morning, 20-round shots would go off. Of course, you were just getting to sleep, and you get woken up from that. The building would literally shake, the windows would shake, the dust would come off the floor; the concussion was that close. And then, of course, the insurgents were rocketing and mortaring us. It was hot there. We pretty much destroyed the whole city. It was nothing but a pile of rubble by the time we left.

We had warned the people. We told them a minimum of three weeks before we went in. We dropped leaflets in. We sent Arabic-speaking people in tell them to get out, that the city was becoming infested with insurgents and that we were going to launch an attack on the city. We didn't tell them when, but it was going to happen. We told them if they wanted to live, they needed to leave, because there would be a day where we would close the city off, and then no one would be allowed to leave and anybody that stayed in the city would be considered a combatant. We warned and warned and warned. I would say 90 percent of the population left. There were a few that stayed.

I saw a horrible TV program after I came back. It was about Fallujah. It was by an Arabic producer, I guess. It was the most blatant propaganda piece I have ever seen in my life. It was interviews talking to people in Fallujah, after it was safe to go in there, talking to the citizens about how terrible the U.S. was destroying their homes, how they couldn't get out of the city, how they were trapped with no food, no water. This was on a regular TV station, a real ultra-liberal channel, called Free Speech TV or something. This was the most blatant propaganda piece on Fallujah. To see this piece, it was basically lies, nothing but lies after lies after lies; interviews with people saying they didn't know it was coming, and they were trapped. That is crap. They were warned over and over and over to get out, get out and get out, but they stayed, and now they blame us. There were civilian casualties out there, but they were people who chose not to leave and got caught in cross fires. We didn't intentionally kill any civilians, but it was a brutal fight. It really was.

There was an incident when a Marine supposedly shot an unarmed insurgent in a mosque, and an embedded cameraman got all of this on video tape. CNN and Fox just aired that video tape over and over. Al Jazeera had a field day with that. Al Jazeera had the best propaganda piece that came out. The Marine was since found not guilty, but the damage that was done was absolutely horrendous.

The part that made me mad was a CNN crew interviewing people at the chow hall. I went up to them and I said, "You guys are missing a good story here." And they said, "What's that?" and I said, "You have been showing on TV, shooting this unarmed insurgent. Al Jazeera has had a field day, but I have not seen one camera crew at the hospital showing pictures of the dozens and dozens of insurgents who our hospital corpsmen and Army medics have come across in the houses of Fallujah who were wounded and gave them medical care and saved their life, and brought them to the hospital for treatment. I have not seen one camera showing us night after night after night saving the lives of the insurgents who were brought to us to whom we gave surgical care. I have not seen the CNN crew filming our American soldiers and sailors standing in the hallway of the hospital, donating their blood in the walking blood bank, to give to the insurgents so that we could save their lives."

I didn't see any of that. Can you imagine if you could get that on Al Jazeera, how that could change the thinking of people? Of course, that would never get on Al Jazeera. We can't even get it on our on TV channels. So he said, "Oh, that sounds like a real good story—what you need to do is to get your public affairs officer to contact us, and we'll be happy to come over and do something like that." They were not interested in showing the good side that our people were doing. They just wanted to show was how much destruction we inflicted on the people of Iraq.

I sometimes think our news media is working for the enemy. I really do. I'm not saying that this shouldn't happen, but they have such a narrow focus they don't want to show the full picture. They only want to show the bad stuff or negative stuff. They don't ever want to show the good stuff. They want to show the pictures of the people screaming, "Get out America. We hate you." They don't want to show the people saying, "God bless America for saving our country." You don't see that. That gets frustrating. We're there to do a mission, to save the guys that get hurt. I'm not getting involved in the political thing, "Should we be there? Should we not be there?" I was there to help save the lives of my heroes. I was there to save people. Should we be in Iraq? We should.

We always focused on the mission. Living conditions were harsh, but we knew we were there for a purpose, and nothing got in our way doing that. I honestly feel from the bottom of my heart that we gave the best medical care that we could have given under the circumstances. Could it have been better? Yeah, if we'd had some better supplies and equipment and stuff, maybe it could have been a better. But we had excellent physicians and nursing staff and corpsmen, they really went above and beyond. I couldn't be happier for that and couldn't be prouder of the people we were working with.

I had to go back to Korean Village after that for the last three or four months. I didn't want to leave Fallujah. I wanted to stay. I said, "I'll stay if you need me. I'd be happy to stay if you need me." After about three weeks, "You gotta get back. You never know, you might be needed." They sent all of us back after about three weeks. We got back in Korean Village the day before Thanksgiving or so. It was nice to have that week in Fallujah. It was the most important thing I have ever done.

LINDA MILLER

Linda Miller began her nursing career at the age of 17 as a licensed practical nurse (LPN). At the age of 39 she returned for her baccalaureate degree in nursing. After a year of nursing experience and time in an intensive care unit, at the age of 46, a single mother and a grandmother of two, she joined the United States Army Nurse Corps reserves.

When I enlisted it was one year post 9/11 and patriotism was at an all time high. I joined for two reasons. One was that I felt it my patriotic duty to assist if I could, and secondly, the monetary gain. I would earn a $10,000 bonus and the U.S. Army would pay $50,000 towards my school loans. Everyone needed critical care nurses, even the Army. Did I know exactly what I was getting into? I am not sure I did.

After enlisting in the reserves and attending drills, my first big Army career step was to attend officer basic training class (OBC). In September of 2003, I went to Fort Sam Houston to what the military refers to as "fork and knife school." It was not the rigorous basic training that the enlisted have to endure. It was three weeks of classes on military etiquette, military protocol and some practical exercises. I learned how to assemble and disassemble a 9mm handgun and an M16 rifle. This was a feat since I have never even held a weapon before. Oh, and by the way, in the Army it is called a weapon and not a gun. I learned to hold my breath and put on a gas mask in less than 60 seconds. I also had to pass a test on litter bearing. The litter-bearing test consisted of groups of four officers. It is your job as a team to carry a litter (stretcher), with a weighted dummy (injured soldier) on it through an obstacle course. First you go over a six-foot wall, then through a narrow aisle, then under barbed wire and finally up a steep grade. We were allowed to practice with our group until we felt ready to take the test.

My team consisted of a male dentist who was small in stature, another nurse that was male and of average build and an ex-ranger that was now a physician's assistant, and he was built like a body builder. Before our practices began I explained to my team that I did not have much upper-body strength and could not get over the wall by myself. It was all right to get assistance from your partners to get over the wall. Not knowing which would be my partner, I practiced with all three to make sure they could get me over the wall. First

103

up was the small-stature dentist. I thought, "Wow, this is going to be a problem because I am no petite lady. I am five foot nine and weigh 180 pounds." Well the dentist did marvelous. He pushed me over with the greatest of ease. Those small men can fool you sometimes at how strong they really are.

Next up was the other RN. He seemed pretty hefty, but as soon as I placed my foot on his leg to use as a ladder to get over the wall, he crumpled. Yikes, I am in trouble. But the instructor, a full-bird colonel, came over and showed him how to stand to withstand my weight. OK, now we got that part straight, the next part was for him to boost me up over the wall. He wouldn't touch me! So I hollered at him, "Grab my butt and push me over the wall. You won't offend me. I cannot get over by myself." We were all laughing, even the colonel.

Last turn was the muscular ex-ranger PA. He practically threw me over the wall. I landed six feet away on the other side of the wall. The colonel instructor peeked around the wall and said, "Are you OK?" I said I was fine, which I was. In fact it was kind of fun. Later I found out that the dentist and the PA had it planned to throw me like that. We all had a good laugh. So then we took the test, managing to get over the wall with our patient, then through a narrow outlet and then under the barbed wire. Oh my! The instructors had soldiers pour old nasty water in the pit, so while we were crawling on our bellies under the wire with this litter in tow, we got thoroughly drenched with mud and dirty water. Then up the steep grade and we were done. We passed!

I continued to work my civilian job as a critical care, open heart nurse and go to my required monthly weekend drills. Then the orders came. I was ordered to report to the 228th CSH (Combat Support Hospital) at Fort Sam Houston for pre–deployment training in September 2004. When I got to Fort Sam Houston, I was housed in the barracks. The barracks consisted of a two-woman room on the fourth floor (no elevators). There was no TV, no computer lines. You shared a shower and bathroom with 12 other women. Sometimes we had hot water, sometimes not. Sometimes we did not have water period. The place was filthy and run down. I would just go on the terrace and cry. My battle buddy/roommate would come out and say, "What is wrong?" I told her I had gone to school, got my degree, was making a nice salary, bought a beautiful home and now I am living in the projects! I lived in these "projects" until we left for Iraq on December 26, 2005.

My pre–deployment training consisted of three-week simulated war games at Fort Polk, Louisiana, warrior training tasks, and SRP (Soldier Readiness Program). The three weeks I was at Fort Polk, all the soldiers (men and women), lived in a large tent that resembled a circus tent. I slept on an Army cot that was far from comfortable. There was no privacy at all. I had to dress and undress under a rain parka — quite a feat since I am five foot nine. Sometimes my butt would be showing while I changed, and my battle buddy would say, "Your butt is showing." I told her, "What do you want me to do? The parka is not long enough." Some of the women dressed and undressed in their sleeping bags, an action that I never could master.

In Fort Polk, Louisiana, the heat was in the 100s, not counting the heat index. It was just plain HOT. Being a nurse in the Army is more than caring for patients. I had to help erect the hospital (tents) in three days. It was rigorous work and in sweltering heat. I came close to heat exhaustion several times. On the third day I was overcome by heat exhaustion, but I wanted to be tough and didn't tell anyone. I marched back to the sleeping tent and was trying to cool off. The tent was air-conditioned but no way could adequately cool this large tent. The next thing I knew they were stripping my clothes off and pouring water on me. I was taxied off to a hospital in a rumbling Army ambulance. I got to the civilian hospital and they gave me three liters of fluid. After several hours of recovering, the nurse came in and said I could go home. I asked her how I was supposed to do that. She said put your clothes on and leave. I said, "Well, all I have is a pair of panties and a bra that is soaking wet, and I live in New Orleans and have no transportation." She asked me if I could contact my unit to come and pick me up. I told her that they dropped me off, that they were somewhere in Fort Polk, and I did not know how to get in touch with them. All the staff thought that I was so crazy to join the Army at my age. They would all come in my room to meet the crazy nurse. A few hours later some enlisted folks from my unit showed up with my uniform and took me back to camp.

Though I was back at camp, I was instructed to stay in quarters for three days. Well, quarters were that large hot tent. By now they had the hospital up and running and there was better air-conditioning, so I decided to walk to the hospital every day. I tried to catch a ride whenever I could because the walk was in the sweltering heat and about a mile's worth of walking. One time I stood at the gate waiting for a vehicle to catch a ride. A Hummer came by, and I asked if I could catch a ride. They said, "Sure, just jump in the back." Well, never ever really having to jump in the back of a Hummer, I was real inexperienced. I couldn't get the back gate open. So I asked the gate guard to assist me in the back. Instead of giving me a knee to step on, he cupped his hands together to boost me up. He boosted before I was ready and he just threw me on my back. My feet kicked up and my boots hit him smack in the mouth. I landed on my back, but I had a water camel on my back so it cushioned my landing. What an experience!

I was feeling better and getting back into the game of things. In JRTC we were all given injury cards. These cards you kept in your upper right pocket, and when instructed to, you opened it up to see what your injuries were. Then you would be treated as if you were injured. Thank goodness I never had to use my injury card, because it said I was shot in the butt!

After three weeks of JRTC, back to San Antonio and Fort Sam Houston we went — a return to more soldier training. In November 2004, I went on a training exercise to Fort Hood in Texas. It was so cold. The tents we lived in were separated by gender, but the air-conditioner was running and it was 30 degrees outside. I have never been so cold in all my life. Again, I slept on an Army cot, which was very uncomfortable. It was just canvas stretched on a metal frame. While at Foot Hood I did simulated war games. I learned how to perform a checkpoint. I learned how to fire my weapon (M16). I learned how to go on a convoy. I learned all about IEDs (improvised explosive devices). All of this training was quite new to me, and none of it did I use when I was in Iraq.

The soldier training done, all the medical clearance done; I was now ready to deploy. I just waited everyday to be told what day we were leaving. While waiting they allowed me to go home for Christmas. That was Christmas, December 2004. We were scheduled to leave for Iraq on December 26, 2004. I had to fly back to Texas from New Orleans on Christmas day. I had my daughter drive me to the airport in New Orleans and then all of a sudden it began to snow. It was snowing so intensely that the airport was closed down — in New Orleans? The airport had plenty of planes but they had no deicing equipment. It just doesn't snow in New Orleans! I was finally able to fly out that night but my luggage got lost. The next day I was in hysterics because they were putting me on a plane to Iraq and I had no luggage. Well, the air line found my luggage but I would not be able to get it until the next day. Thank God that an NCO went and got my luggage the next day and sent it on the second plane going to Iraq. Whew! What a mess. My luggage met up with me in Kuwait the next day when the second part of our unit arrived.

After a short stop in Germany, we were flown to Kuwait. Welcome to the Middle East — areas of the world for a soldier where there are no TVs, no cell phones, no private baths or showers, and no transportation to save your two feet. We were housed in tents again. Thank goodness we were separated by gender, and unlike Fort Hood, the air-conditioners and heaters worked perfectly to keep us comfortable.

The 228th was a small reserve unit, so the Army brought in hundreds of soldiers from around the world. Some were active duty, some were reservists. One half of my unit was tasked to go to Mosul, Iraq, and the other half was tasked to go to Tikrit, Iraq. I was assigned to go to Tikrit. I was in Kuwait, awaiting movement orders. Then I and 14 other critical care nurses were tasked to go work in an Air Force Hospital in Balad, Iraq.

Camp Virginia in Kuwait was a large sprawling FOB (forward operating base). It was all dirt, sand and rocks. I never saw any grass or foliage. I was in Camp Virginia for about a week, then I was flown, via a large cargo plane, to Balad, Iraq. Riding the cargo plane was quite an experience. You sit on a hard

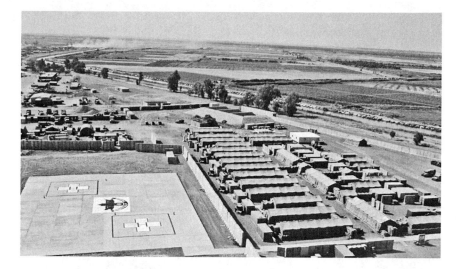

Camp Hospital in Balad, Iraq

bench. There is no heating or air-conditioning. So, when you were on land you were hot, and then when you were up in the air it was freezing cold. Four hours is a long time to sit on a hard bench. The bathroom was just a bucket with a curtain around it. Each leg of this journey seemed to be more primitive than the last.

Alas, I arrived in Balad, Iraq. Again, there was no foliage to be seen. Just sand, sand, sand, and more sand. I was bussed to the hospital. There I was introduced to the 332 EMDG Air Force administrative staff and given housing. I was given a two-woman room to stay in, which was a third of a trailer. My bathroom was the port-a-john about 100 yards from my room. My shower was a community shower about 500 yards from my room. The room consisted of a single bed (YAHOO), no more cots. It also had a foot locker and a bedside table. The trailers were in areas that were surrounded by cement walls and bunkers. The trailers themselves were surrounded by sandbags about five feet high. The cement walls, bunkers and sandbags were to protect you from mortar attacks, which occurred on a weekly basis.

The Air Force personnel only do four-month rotations, compared to the Army's twelve-month rotations. So soon after arriving I was able to buy some amenities from a departing Air Force soldier. I bought a wet vac, a microwave, a small refrigerator, a fan, some rugs, and a much-needed converter. The electricity in the housing area was 220, unlike in America which is 110. So in order to run anything American made, you had to have a converter. Each room had a heater/air-conditioner which worked superbly to keep me comfortable.

There was a short rainy season in Iraq. The sand turned to thick muck that stuck on your boots three inches thick. Cleaning the water and mud in the hospital was a constant battle. After the short period of rain, there was no spring, just — BAM — summer. The hottest it got when I was there was 138 degree Fahrenheit. It reminded me a lot of the beach, sandy and bright with a little wind. Due to the heat, water stations were scattered throughout Camp Anaconda. Water stations consisted of dozens of boxes of bottled water. Bottled water is the only water we drank; all other water was not potable.

I began working at the hospital and soon found out what it is to work in a war. The 332 EMDG was a multi-coalition hospital, and I had the opportunity to work with the U.S. Air Force, U.S. Navy and the Australian Army. I worked 12–14 hours a day seven days a week. I rarely had a day off. And when I had a day off, I was so exhausted all I could do was sleep. The Balad Hospital was in Camp Anaconda. This, for an FOB, had quite a few amenities. There was a Burger King, Pizza Hut, PX, swimming pool, and theater. I rarely took advantage of these amenities because of my work schedule, and I was just too tired.

We tried to lighten up whenever we could to try to relieve the stress of constant working. One day we took some balloons and made a patient and equipped him with all the accessories of an ICU patient — ETT tube, feeding tube, VP drains, etc. We all had a ball with it and thought it was good light humor, but the flight commander didn't agree. He had us disassemble it immediately. My most valued morale booster was mail call. Americans would send us so many packages it was astounding. My daughter sent a small portable ice machine. That was the greatest mail I received while I was over there. I placed it in the hospital so we could use it for ourselves and also for our patients.

The critical care unit of the hospital had three wards— one ward for Americans, one ward for Iraqis and one ward was for overflow. Along with critical care patients we also did recovery

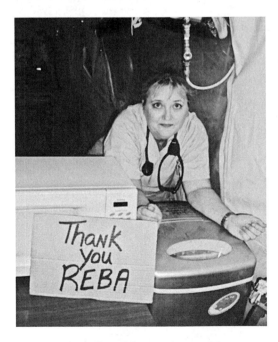

Linda Miller with camp ice machine.

of surgical patients. Each ward consisted of ten beds. The beds were similar to Army cots that were on wire frames at waist level. The foot and head were able to lift up. We placed orange mattresses on them for added comfort. The beds were very narrow, about three feet wide. These narrow beds were extremely difficult for patient turning. There were no safety rails. We cared for patients in a very small, confined area, cramped with critical care equipment like ventilators, suction machines, etc. Nursing was a challenge.

I received patients from other FOBs or directly from the field. They always arrived via a helicopter. The helipad was directly adjacent to the hospital. The only identification the patients had was what was written on them. If they were American they would have a trauma number or the last four digits of their social security number written on their chest. Because communication at war was difficult, patients often arrived with a written summary on them.

I don't think any of the nurses were aware of the extent of the traumas that we would receive or care for. The 332 EMDG hospital was the only hospital in the field that I am aware of that had neurosurgeons. We cared for hundreds of brain injury patients. Our supplies were always limited. We often would run out of items and have to improvise. We only had colostomy bags and no urostomy bags, so I developed my own wound drainage bag, using a colostomy bag and an irrigation syringe. Linen was always short. The patients were extremely high acuity traumas.

The American soldiers were always separated from the other patients. Usually within 12 hours of receiving them they were packaged up, critical care equipment and all, and flown to Germany. The Air Force team of doctors, nurses and respiratory therapist would care for and escort the American patients on the plane for the six-hour flight to Germany. The team was called the CCAT team, and they often brought the nurses chocolate and Cinnabons, which we devoured.

The Iraqi patients were another issue. We found ourselves stuck taking care of them for months. Our CSH frequently was turned into a long-term care facility. After their initial care there was no place for us to send them. Iraq has a very poor medical system, and definitely had no long-term care facilities. We were frequently forced to discharge Iraqi patients home. We instructed the family as best we could on how to care for them. The doctors would insert a very large bore gastric tube for feedings. Iraqi families had no commercial tube feedings or blenders. They fed their family members mashed food via the feeding tube. But the greatest thing I learned medically about the Iraqi culture is that they are very resilient and that they have a very high tolerance for pain. I cared for Iraqi patients with gunshot wounds to the head and explosive wounds to their abdomens. In the United States a patient like that rarely made it to the emergency room, much less survived. But the Iraqi patients always surprised me with their resilience. I remember two specific occasions where Iraqis had head injuries and were placed in the expectant area. The expectant area is where dying patients were placed. A nurse and a clergyman would monitor them and keep them sedated and comfortable until they expired. But these two Iraqis did not die. When the paralytic wore off, they were getting up off the stretcher. Whoops, better rethink this situation and do some brain surgery. Both patients survived.

I cared for all kinds of patients. Not only did I care for American and coalition soldiers, I also cared for Iraqis (good and bad), contract workers and children. All of these patients received the equal amount of care.

Prisoners were always blindfolded and had a guard. I never knew what they did, but sometimes we knew if they were high-level security. The prisoners were not allowed to speak unless we spoke to them. Many would come in and surprisingly spoke a small bit of English. Several of them would say, "I you friend." I would ask them, "If you are our friend, why are you trying to kill us?" Once the prisoners were treated and stable, they were transferred to Abu Ghraib (prison), where there was a hospital. We always had interpreters available for our Iraqi population. Arabic is a hard language but I did learn a few words like "pain" and "take a deep breath." I was astonished to learn that there are so many ways to communicate other than speaking.

Caring for contract workers was another issue. Contractors would subcontract several times, so even though the patient said they worked for KBR (the main American contractor there) that was not the case. Then we had to find out what country they were from, try to find their passports and try to get a facility in their country to accept them — not an easy task which took several weeks to accomplish.

One type of patient that none of us were prepared for was the infants and children. Some were injured in war activities, but some just showed up at the gate for care. It was the commander's decision to accept a non–battle related patient. It was difficult to turn away the kids, so we often did charity cases. One reason is that it established a good relation with the community, and it was just hard to turn a head to those little cuties. None of us were experienced with children. We constantly were reading in reference books we had brought to assist us. We would take turns taking care of the kids because it was so difficult. On election day the hospital birthed a baby. There was a curfew in effect, and the mom got stuck at the hospital and went into labor. It was exciting, because you don't deploy OB doctors to war, so we improvised the best we could. It all worked out well and mama and baby were fine. It was very grueling to care for the infants and children, but the families we so grateful to us they would kiss us and say, "Thanks to Allah."

I was assaulted three times while I was in Iraq. The first time I was outside the hospital smoking a cigarette in the bunker, when a very young Iraqi National Guard walked up to me. I thought he was going to ask for a cigarette, but instead he began to speak to me in broken English. He would point at things and say the name in Arabic and then ask me to say the name in English. We did this for my name, my boots, my pants, etc. Then he touched my breast and asked what it was in English. He then pointed to my genitals and asked what it was called. I had a boot knife and I pulled it on him, and told him if he touched me again I would slice him open. He was arrested and exiled from the hospital by the commander.

The second occurrence happened with a Jordanian patient. He spoke very good English and came in with chest pain. I was starting an IV on him and he stuck his toe in my crotch. He was immediately transferred out of the hospital.

The third occurrence was with another patient of mine that was an Iraqi policeman. He had brain surgery and his eyes were swollen shut. I had him sitting in a chair, feeding him, when he began to feel my face. He then grabbed me by my neck and forced my face in his crotch. I was screaming for someone to help me, but no one could hear over the loud noises in the unit. Then my OIC (officer in charge), a LTC, looked up from her desk and said, "Miller, what are you doing." My coworkers helped free me, and we transferred him to the ward. There was a lot of sexual inappropriateness with Iraqi patients. It was something that we constantly were cautious of. Being a blonde is your worst enemy in this culture.

Throughout the year we were constantly visited by generals from the Army and the Air Force. They showed great concern for both the injured Americans and all the staff. It was great to shake the hand of a general and for them to acknowledge our hard work.

While I was in Iraq, my daughter birthed my third grandchild, and my home was destroyed by hurricane Katrina. I had to deal with the issues of war along with home-front issues. I have been away from home now for almost two years, a long time to be away from my loved ones.

I returned from Iraq in December 2005. Since I returned I have been receiving medical treatment for injuries sustained in Iraq. The parts of my body that were affected by working for a year in war are: my ears, my right shoulder, both knees, both ankles, depression and post–traumatic stress. I am dealing with these issues and I am hoping that I can be able to return home soon. My unit is scheduled to return to Iraq in November 2007.

KAREN
NIEMANTSVERDRIET-McDONALD

Many nurses who have served and continue to serve during the Persian Gulf Wars serve at sites other than the battle front. These are courageous nurses with a great deal of experience. They make important decisions while serving their fellow serviceman on humanitarian missions. These decisions have great impact on the lives of those they serve.

I graduated from Washington State University in nursing in December of 1984. Remember this was back in the 1980s. It was back when nurses were still pretty subservient to doctors. Doctors were the ones that brought in the finances and the patients. Without the physicians nurses didn't have employment. I was assisting in a procedure when a neurosurgeon was putting a bolt into somebody's head. He touched something and contaminated his sterile field. I asked him if he would like to have a new pair of gloves. This was a Catholic hospital in which I was doing my nursing training. I was called down to the sister's office and was told if I ever talked back to a physician again or embarrassed him in front of a patient's family, I would no longer be allowed to work in that facility. I just kind of looked at them and said, "Do you know I was just trying to prevent an infection?" That didn't matter. Remember, back then doctors really were the ones that brought in the money, so you didn't make the doctors mad.

I can remember another time I was charting. We had these little cubicles where we could chart. I can remember I was just sitting in my own little cubicle, charting. A physician came and he took the chart so he could read the name on the front of it. He didn't say anything to me. He just flipped it, pinching my fingers and then proceeded to pull the chart away. He took my pen out of my hand, turned my chair around and told me to go get coffee. I took the chart back, took my pen back, told him getting coffee wasn't in my job description. I was down in the sister's office again.

So, then I decided, well maybe, you know my dad was military and I know they don't treat people like that. You have rank. You have a position. You have authority. You work one-on-one, collegially with the physicians. So, I walked that day right down to the recruiter's office and said, "OK, you know

112

what, I think it's going to be best if I join the Navy." I was still in nursing training, so they did not fire me, but they wouldn't let me go back onto that ward because that physician was mad that I didn't go get him coffee or let him have a chart and a pen. If he would have said, "Please," I would have done anything.

Karen served at San Diego Naval Medical Center and at the Naval Hospital in Naples, Italy, in the ICU. She served in the air evac system taking patients from Italy to Landstuhl, Germany. She thought she would be deployed from Italy to the Gulf War.

I was stationed over in Naples, Italy, when were on our very first Gulf War. My husband went over as a JAG Corps Officer, mainly for anything that would happen in international waters because he was an international JAG officer. That was his specialty. We were also on standby to go over and put the very first fleet hospital up. I have to tell you I almost got out at that point because I had an eight-month-old infant. She was on one plane on the tarmac pointed towards the states and I was in another plane pointed towards Rota, Spain, where we were going to go pick up the fleet hospital and go on over to Iraq. My husband was in Iraq and I couldn't talk to him. At the very last minute the Gulf War didn't have as many casualties as they thought, so they stood us down and had us on a 24-hour watch for several weeks, but we didn't have to go anywhere. If they had told me I had to go, I would have had to go. My baby would have had to go home to my mom. Actually, our commanding officer's wife was on that plane with probably three children. Mine was the youngest, but she had a five-year-old. Again, people like me who were either single parents or they were dual active duty were being mobilized on short notice. Thank God, she was a lovely, lovely woman and she knew that if that was ever going to happen, she was going to take quite a few children home.

That's what we all have to do whenever there is dual military. You have to have a backup. You have to have a family care plan in case the both of you have to be gone at the same time. It's also in case both of us get in an automobile accident and then you're left with what do you do with these kids. We have to have it documented. In some ways it's very good. It made you think about financial issues such as having money for a standby plane ticket and whether someone else would be able to manage the finances if you couldn't.

Karen finished up the first Gulf War in Naples, went back to Charleston, South Carolina, to Charleston Naval Hospital and back to the ICU and to the newborn nursery. She taught corpsmen and oriented new nurses to their naval roles. She returned to get her master's degree in nursing at the University of San Diego. She became a family nurse practitioner and served in Japan and Hawaii.

By this time the second Gulf conflict was going on. From Hawaii I was selected to be one of the four positions where I was a nurse to the fleet. It was in San Diego. I belonged to Balboa Naval Medical Center San Diego, but I was added to the staff of commander, Amphibious Group 3. This group included all of the amphibious assault ships that carried the Marines to wherever they need to go; the Germantown, the Boxer, Pearl Harbor, Rushmore, Lassen, Ogden. I served on all those ships. I served wherever the fleet needed any type of a primary care provider.

The way I first got my foot in the door with the ships was because there are now a lot of women on the ships. There are not so many nurses on board the ships if you look at the sheer number of females attached to a ship doing the other jobs, the real line jobs, like the Boxer. The Boxer had at least 55 percent of the entire sailors onboard being female. If you think of all those women who were in their prime childbearing years, stressed, away from family, and sexually active; that's a whole population that needs care that they feel safe in getting. When you're stationed on a ship, the corpsmen that you eat and drink and go out and see the area with are also the same ones giving you your care. Many of them, as patients, feared for their privacy. Whether it was a founded or unfounded fear, they really feared for their privacy — especially the people who were more senior and had to interact with the single medical officers stationed on each ship. They didn't want to be sitting next to them in the ward room having dinner every night or sitting next to them at whatever disaster station they had to go to, if they knew everything about them. If they had an STD and it was because they slept with this person, obviously the physician is going to know who those two people are. It was really putting the women at risk.

I went on those ships, especially before they were going to be deployed for a sixth-month time period, to get all of the women's readiness up. I did all their well-women's exams, got them on birth control, and took care of whatever they needed including some of the ones that they were afraid to talk about, whether it's a breast reduction or their acne or their genital warts. Whatever they needed me to take care of, I would do. In the morning when we had sick call, I would teach the corpsmen how to do sick call screeners and take care of their own population. When they do get called up to war, they knew the basics; how to do a good knee exam or back exam, how to take care of somebody who's dehydrated or common colds, and what are the common medicines that you would carry with you backpack. That's all our job, too, when you go out on ships.

When I first started I would only go out with them prior to them going away. Before, the person who was in my job would just see them if they were tied up to the pier. My goal would be to go underway with them for a short period of time, anywhere from three days to two weeks. While the population was captive, they can't be leaving the ship or avoiding these exams, I could see them. This was when they would go away for their six months, going to Iraq or wherever they were going to play their war games at that time. When they were coming home I would usually meet them 10 to 14 days outside of San Diego. I would either fly to Hawaii or fly to the coast that they were coming by, and I would sail home with them, again to take care of all their female readiness issues before they set foot back on ground. If the ship got turned around and in a short time got sent out again, they were back up with their readiness levels.

There are four family nurse practitioners attached to the fleet. Each of us did things a little bit differently. It depended on what the COs and the medical officers on the ships would allow me to do. You have to kind of get in with them. After I started going out, I realized that we could fill in for the primary care providers permanently attached to the ship. If the Boxer's physician wanted to go on leave, rather than leave the ship with no medical assets, the ship would let me fly out and be the medical officer for that period of time. On one of the small ships, the Ogden, the physician wanted to get married. He didn't have anybody to fill in. They were actually going to cancel his wedding and honeymoon. I put my hand up and said, "I'll go and be your medical officer."

So we started getting out as the medical officers on board the ships. Not full time, just filling in where they needed us. Then we figured out when you go on some of these missions, we needed to have augmented stuff. We needed to have more providers—like the Boxer went out for a period of I think two months and they just realized that one person wasn't going to be enough for the crew needs since they were being turned around and being redeployed. There were a lot of mental health issues. There was a lot of stuff that we would wait and wait and wait until we got back in and those issues really needed to be dealt with. So they brought me underway and I actually floated with them for two months, though not a whole six-month deployment in Iraq. I did go out with them doing many southern California operations. I got to the ships by helicopter. I would have to fly to whatever coastline was close to the ship. I could go by any sort of hopper or civilian aircraft and they would pay me to go. Sometimes I would even go to from the Boxer to one of the smaller ships on a helicopter. I actually had to kind of figure out what would work with the medical officers and say, "OK, I need to get to your ship on this date. Here's my information. Here's my cell phone. Tell me where you want me to pick up the helo and how I'm going to get there." Sometimes I'd have to leapfrog different ships to get to that final one. It was kind of me working with the medical department. They would work with their ops officers to figure out how they were going to get me out there. Of course, I had to get permission from the commanding officer to get onboard. I was credentialed by service forces in San Diego, so I could go really on any gray hull that I wanted to as long as they knew where I was going. I had to just let them know who I was seeing and what I was doing. They were very supportive and it was really fun.

I was doing that up until the day of the tsunami, the 26th of December 2005. On the 28th I got a phone call that said, "You always keep your bags packed, right, because you go to ships daily right?" I was like: "Yes." "Want to go on the Mercy?" So we left on the 5th of January of 2006, and I went on nearly a six-month deployment with the USNS Mercy. I went out on the Mercy as the assistant director of nursing and quickly fell into being the liaison officer ashore. I was the one who had to go into these big tents or whatever mobile hospital was put up or the remaining structure that we moved into. I was the one that triaged the Indonesian patients and decided, "You can go to the Mercy. We can take care of you. I'm sorry you're too sick for the time period that we're going to be here to help you."

I did a lot of that liaison work with the existing cultural hospital or medical assets that were still remaining, plus a lot of the United Nations response teams that came over; USAID, Singapore Hospital, Mercy Aid. I can't think of them all right now, but they're just everywhere. We were working with Project Hope aboard the ship. We had everybody in the world that had anything over there. We had the Germans and Australians that were there. We had a Spanish ship that was off the coast there plus the Mercy was off the coast. We did not have any of the actual waterfront. Piers were gone and ships and boats were gone because of the tsunami. The only transportation we had was a helicopter. There was a helicopter support ship that was left behind with the Mercy.

As soon as we came into the waters, the Lincoln battle group had to leave because Lincoln battle group was more of the armored side and the Indonesians didn't want them there. They wanted them out of those waters. Indonesia and Banda Aceh, where we were stationed, was closed to any foreigners at all. It was a very, very, very poor area. They only took the military help, especially the American military. This is a Muslim country and they didn't like us. They didn't really want to even have our people there, but they couldn't ignore this catastrophe that had happened. So they agreed that they would allow the Mercy to come in, but the Lincoln battle group had to be out before the Mercy could come in.

This was the first time the Mercy had been deployed in 15 years. We had to do a lot of: How do we make things work? How are we going to get supplies? This is going to be a humanitarian mission and we have never done it when it's been solely with the helicopter. This was actually a ship that was supposed to take care of wartime people, which were usually young, healthy males. We didn't have the pediatric size endotracheal tubes or IVs. We didn't own a crib. We did have one baby delivery table that had an infant warmer, and we got a bilirubin light before we left. But stuff like high chairs, play pens, a bed with real sides on it were nonexistent. We had some stuff, but again we're not looking for really, really sick intubated people, people who were already baseline malnourished. We didn't get on site until a month after the tsunami, so there were infected wounds. We learned a lot. We changed the supplies the ship is carrying. We now have a humanitarian AMAL and stuff that we had all put together, and we have maintained so that when this happens, we will have the right stuff when we get there.

We were coming home from Banda Aceh and we were stopping at a few other places in the Indonesia allure. Then we stopped at Bali. At that point they had an 8.5 earthquake that happened in Nias Island. We turned around at the request of the Indonesian government and went to respond to them in Nias. Because we were close this time, we were one of the first people that were actually on site. Australian Aid was wonderful. They were there. The UN was there with their helicopters because this earthquake had taken most of the roads that were very scant anyhow. They were actually going and flying to these different helipads that were kind of created and bringing out the very injured. There were a lot more spinal cord injuries, a lot more fractures, a lot more acutely ill patients because we got there so fast. So we stayed there for I think 28 days and then we were told we had to be out by a certain time. We got everybody as healthy as we could, and we helped to rebuild the existing hospital. We had structural engineers on board, and they determined what parts of the hospital were still serviceable. We helped by donating of a lot of mattresses and stuff.

We left from Nias to go to Papua, New Guinea. At Papua, New Guinea they did have one major city that was doing pretty well on its own. They actually wanted us to do more of a JCAHO survey and help them with some of their internal processes. We helped them set up some computer networks and some more complicated surgical cases that they didn't either have all of the surgical instruments or maybe all the talent to do. We worked side by side in their hospital.

I didn't actually stay in New Guinea. There was an erupting island, a volcano that was erupting that caused all of those people from that island to be displaced and put in IDP camps (internally displaced persons camps). I actually was selected to be the OIC to go and provide outreach dental, medical and preventive care. This included Seabees constructing some semi-permanent structures. We also had preventive health and preventive medicine that would go out and spray and make sure people weren't going to get ill from anything that could be prevented. There were a lot of mosquitoes, a lot of malaria, etc. People were coming from a place that was malaria free to a place where now there was malaria indigenous to that area. So we were trying to put up a lot of bed nets and teaching them how to dip their bed nets. We were teaching them how to use them for something appropriate, instead of using them to dry their clothes on. We taught them how to dip every 3–6 months, whatever it turned out they needed to do. We bought them the buckets and the stuff to do that, taught them how to store it. We gave them many medical supplies and immunized all of the children and the moms. We passed out more glasses than I can remember to anybody who had age-related changes in their eyes. We did that free. We pulled teeth if they needed to be pulled.

People over there had things we don't even think about dying from anymore. I had never seen active cases of tetanus until I went over there. We did a lot of tetanus immunizations. They walk around barefoot. There are all these pieces of metal stuff lying around, and they can get infected pretty easily. So we did a lot of great things in these three outreach camps that we went to. We took care of everybody in all the camps, but we only visited three and they came to us on different days. It's just wonderful memories to know that we helped them. They were just so great.

We had people lined up for miles. We brought in water for them that they needed. We airlifted in a lot of things that they needed. The government of Papua, New Guinea really didn't do much for these people. These were not people that they took care of, that they really would have been responsible for. These people were between a rock and a hard place. You know they were stuck here because their island has hot lava flowing on it, but they had to leave every part of their possessions including their fishing boat, which was their only way of livelihood. Now they're relying on a country that really doesn't want to give them a buck. So we provide a lot of great care for them. They were just lovely, lovely people. They would eventually go home if the volcano would quiet down. I think they got to go home once and they got evacuated out again.

We were trying to work with Papua, New Guinea to see if maybe there was a way we could get those fishing boats back over. Then they could actually at least make a living for themselves, even though they were on a different coast. They didn't have the money to buy another fishing boat or all the supplies that were still in existence on their own fishing boats. The volcano had not gone down to where the fishing villages were. We were trying to work some of that stuff out. Again, it's one of those political things. We can do what we could do on that day. We had worked with people who were working with those communities already, so we were leaving some things. At least we left all the information for the people who were going to follow on after us; which kids had been immunized and when they were due the next ones, etc.

I got off the Mercy in June 2005. I think in July 2005 I went back out on the Boxer. I counted up and I think I was gone about 400 days in two years. My husband was great. He had actually been deployed to Iraq and had been home about 60 days when I got the call up to go to the tsunami. Since I had been going out so much, my parents had come to help us out. My kids were a little bit older then. I had a freshman and sophomore in high school at that point. My son was sixth and seventh grade. They were great, great kids, very self reliant. When my husband came back from Iraq, he saw how much I was being deployed and what was going on. He said, "OK, that's enough. I'm at 20, I'm getting out."

He retired and then we got orders up to San Diego. It was very good. He was extremely supportive of everything I did. I can tell you there's no way I could have reached my rank in the Navy and been able to hold the positions of responsibility without the teamwork that we did together. On some days he's more the mom than I am, and some days I'm more of the mom than he is. It just depends. The person who's keeping the house together everyday just changes. My parents actually live in Washington state. We always just had an open plane ticket, so if I ever needed them, I could call one or both of them to come out and help.

The Navy family really doesn't mean just blood. If you were like: "Oh goodness, I was supposed to be home and now we're turning around to go back to Nias." We were on our way home on the Mercy and we turned around. So my kids were all like: "What do you mean? Dad's not here now and you're supposed to be." "That's OK, you know, we got friends. You can stay with these friend for four days and Grandma will be right there." My kids have been fabulous with all this. We moved up, my daughter was a junior. I just went to the open house and the teachers said, "We didn't even know she was new. She had so many friends and she's really outgoing."

Catholic is the faith that we claim and go to. Having this faith I think has definitely helped. One thing about being on the ships, even though you are around 5,000 people, you can still feel pretty socially isolated. Being able to go to mass on the ships and finding people and singing together as a group really helped with the isolation. Obviously, it was something really special. Most of the chapels are kind of part of the flight area or extra bulkhead space. You just found your faith and your community wherever you went, especially on the Mercy when we would be so exhausted. Sundays were the only day that we didn't fly. We would be so mentally exhausted and giving, giving, giving. Sometimes just taking a time to be together doing something that was very ritualistic to us was very comforting to us—singing together, praying together, being with each other, and listening to each other as we kind of missed the things that are very materialistic.

We missed our families. I missed having my own room, because we would sleep in a room that had six other officers in it. It was like back in dormitory time. I missed having my own bathroom. I have to take a shower with 15 of my closest friends. We realized by the end how materialistic we started out. We definitely felt by the end of that, as Americans, we are pretty spoiled — believing that the most toys win. That probably isn't at all we need to do. We actually would tell people that they taught us more than we taught them. They taught us that family was the most important thing and their faith was the most important thing.

I can remember when we were over in Indonesia there were many, many people that did not make it. One of my jobs was every afternoon I had to drive out to the airfields to talk to the brigadier general of the Indonesian Army and Air Force, to have airspace the next day to fly my helicopters in. That was part of my job. Every day I would kind of see this open field that looked like it had just been tilled and leveled, and every day it would kind of change its size. One day they were putting up this sign, and I talked to my interpreter and my driver and said, "I would like to stop. I want to know what the sign says." My interpreter did his best to try and talk me out of it. I said, "No, I really, really want to know what this is." So he takes me out and he's explaining to me what was written on this very small, maybe 12 by 18 inch space. It was a very, very small sign. It turns out this is a mass gravesite. This is where everyone who didn't make it was being buried. These were the bodies that weren't swept away. Everyday that you would go along you would see that there were these orange sticks that were put into the ground. That just told you that's where a body was. When we sent the people to go and retrieve the bodies in the body bags, this is where they brought them everyday and they buried them. As they unearthed things or as the water receded or as it evaporated, we were finding more people everyday. So this is where they were burying them. I said, "Oh, here's all this open space." I said, "So, are they going to make a memorial park or are they going to come up with something? Do you have a planning group? What are they doing?" I was talking to him about in America when the Twin Towers went down we had this big hole. It's like a big sore to us in America. We want to build something so we never forget. And he looked at me and he said, "Why would we ever build anything that would bring so much sadness to everyone who visits. This will be homes." It's just a totally different way of thinking.

We changed how we view the world by the Mercy deployment and by many of my deployments. It changed what I thought was really important. My car and the square footage of my house are not important. Family is important. Faith is important. Family doesn't have to mean just blood family. A lot of times when these people talk about their aunties and their uncles, they're not blood related. It's family that's there for them, because you can lose your whole family in a minute. And they did. I think I have been able to communicate to my family and friends what I have experienced because we had the digital cameras there. We could take a lot of pictures that we could sift through. I can tell you I probably didn't look at my digital pictures for about three months, because it hurt me to remember again.

I had to leave so many of those people we wanted to help. We couldn't help them. A lot of these people had chronic diseases. They had cancer that was everywhere. Stuff that we would find as a small one-centimeter mass was a seven-inch mass. A lot of what we did was not related to the tsunami, but existing chronic disease. Because we were free medical care in a place where there was a fee for service, people were flying in from other cities in Indonesia to get this free care. That's how expensive medical care is. I think it was very, very hard.

My children hated it when they'd come up to me and say, "Mom, I NEED 20 bucks today." And I'd be like: "You don't NEED anything. You have more in your life then every single child I ever saw over in Indonesia. You need nothing. Now if you would say I would like to have, we can have this discussion. But, you need to realize that the more toys you have doesn't mean that you're the best." So I think that was probably the one thing we did talk about. My children were very mad for a while, but I think once they sat down and saw some of the stuff that we had seen and what we were talking about, they were much better.

SANDY PETERS

It took Sandy Peters until the age of 35 to decide that nursing was the right career for her. After working in financial business until that time, she decided to go back to nursing school. She said, "I would go to work and do my job and it felt like everybody just wanted more. Everyone was greedy and it was all about money. I always wanted to get back into the medical profession where I felt like I was part of something worthwhile. I wanted to help people regain something of their lives."

Sandy said of her mother, "So many times I wanted to quit nursing school because it was such a challenge with all the kids. If it hadn't been for my mother, I would have quit numerous times. She is my hero. I would threaten to get out of nursing and she would say, 'You're not going to quit this. You are going to do this. Let's sit down and study. You'll get through it. You can do this.' She just kept me on track. Moms are great that way. They believe in you even when you can't."

After graduation Sandy worked transitional care, diabetic care, oncology, ICU and recovery room. Feeling the need to do some type of service (as though nursing service wasn't enough) she went to Thailand with Operation Smile. The experience lead her to thinking about joining the military. That decision lead her to making major decisions that affected the lives of peers and patients alike.

My dad had been in the military and had been in during World War II. While I was in nursing school, I kind of played around with the idea of joining the military. When I came back from Operation Smile, I decided to look into it. I checked into the Navy. I was 42 and the Navy thought I was too old. I said, "You guys are crying for nurses. I'm not too old. I am very healthy. I was a gymnast when I was younger." I probably could have run circles around a lot of them. I didn't join while I was in college because I just didn't want to go through the basic training. If you join afterwards you join as an officer. You do basic, but a different kind. I kept playing around with the idea.

Finally, one of the Army recruiters said, "Oh sure, we would love to have you." By that time, because of my experience in bone marrow transplant and my experience in PACU with art lines and ventilators, I was able to get the 8A designator, which is for ICU. I had also taken the intensive care courses at LDS Hospital. That is how I got into the intensive care. I found myself hovering close to that "live on the edge, exciting, think on your feet "type of nursing." I kind of veered toward the intensive care. Besides, I love to camp. I'm not afraid of the dirt. They told me right up front, "If you are afraid of being dirty or being out in the wild, afraid of sleeping in a tent, this is not for you." My parents spent a lot of time with us outside. I'm not high maintenance that way.

Fort Douglas in Salt Lake City was where we drilled. Nobody told me how to wear my uniform or tuck my laces in or how to wear my hat. I showed up with my uniform out of regulation on the first day. But the enlisted people were so nice. They would come up and whisper, "Ma'am, you need to tuck your laces in your boots." They were really respectful. I thought how awesome those young people were. They respected me and helped and mentored me. I am just this old lady joining the military. They were so kind and making me look okay. That is actually how I got into the military.

I joined for a couple of reasons. I thought I could get the same feeling of fulfillment from being in the military that I had with the trip to Thailand. I couldn't explain to anyone how that felt to have done the mission in Thailand, to have seen those children and seen what a difference it made for me to go over there and take care of them for 20 or 30 minutes while they woke up from their surgery. I could play with them or hold them and watch how their lives changed because of that. I wasn't even able to explain this to my family. I tried, but they didn't get it. I think most people don't get it. You have to feel it.

The recruiter also talked to me about furthering my education. It was kind of a little bone that they threw me, even though I had already considered going on. I had always wanted to get my master's degree. I have always tried to make myself a better person. I was thinking I could go into trauma. I could get my master's degree in acute care and go into trauma. The Army was looking for acute care nurse practitioners. The Army did help me. They helped me with some of my student loans. There is a ceiling on how much the Army can give you. I went to the University of Utah for my master's degree.

As an ICU nurse I did a couple of small missions with the Army. I went to Germany and worked in a clinic. I did immunizations. I was always volunteering to do the humanitarian missions. Usually they last about two weeks. Our unit had been deployed with Desert Storm to Germany. They were there about three months. That was just prior to when I joined. Then the second Gulf War broke out and we received our alert orders in early 2005.

When all the stuff started happening in the Gulf, I had a feeling I would be going. We were one of the largest combat support hospitals in the United States. We were completely up to speed. We had just passed off all the certifications. My husband and I had talked about me being deployed. He said they would never take me. I knew he was worried and probably not prepared for me to go. He was probably not really receptive to the idea. He didn't have a problem when I joined. I know that he had always wanted to be in the military, but he never could because of some issues with his vision. I kept saying, "You know, this might happen." At this point most of my kids were moved out. My oldest son and my twins still lived at home. We finally got our alert orders and I said, "This means I'm going."

There was no date on the orders. They said get ready. Sometimes they give you three days. Sometimes they give you three or four months. Sometimes it is longer than that depending on where they are going to send you. When we talked to our unit, they first said we were going to Iraq. Then they changed it to Germany, back to Iraq, back to Germany. They did this four times. We never really knew where we were going until late November, when they finally gave us our orders. They were for 18 months in Germany

We weren't even supposed to deploy until January 5. But I was advanced party because I was the mobilization officer. I was in charge of taking 245 soldiers to Germany. I hadn't ever done that before. I knew how to be a nurse, but I had never mobilized 245 soldiers before. I practiced at it in the unit. That was one of the things I was learning. I wanted to learn other things besides nursing. I wanted to be a good officer and take care of my troops. It was very interesting to take all those people and deal with the emotions and other problems. There were six officers. I was the mobilization officer. There was also a commander, a chief of nursing service, personnel, etc. I was to oversee the whole mobilization, and then I had a team that branched out to do their parts. At this point I was a captain and 50 years old.

It was very challenging. Most of the soldiers that were deployed wanted to go and do their part. This was what they had trained for. They were excited. But then we had soldiers that thought, "I never knew this could happen. I don't want to go over there. I am going to lose this, that and the other." I can say that most of our unit was ready and strong. I don't think they were really prepared for what they would encounter and deal with. The war had been going on for a while. Combat support hospitals were rotating through. I just don't think anybody really thought they would pick little old Utah and send our combat support hospital.

What they didn't realize was how big our hospital was and how much they needed a hospital that would fill 245 spaces. We had actually pulled a few people from Montana and Idaho. One fellow came from New Jersey. For the bulk of it, we had enough soldiers. When we got to Germany we were 80 percent of the staff of the hospital. They had their administrative people there, but we staffed everything in the hospital, including the dining room. The administrative people were active duty, mostly Air Force because we were close to Ramstein Air Force Base.

Emotions were very high. It was sad sometimes for many of the women. As soon as some of them got deployed, their husbands left them. Within the first two or three months we were over there, I know of five women who found themselves single. Their husbands had cleaned them out financially or taken their children. Deployments do really weird things to people. I don't think the spouses are prepared for what is going on. When I went over my husband wouldn't talk to me for seven months. Before I left we were talking. Just before I left he got angry at me. It was some really silly, off-the-wall communication issue. He wouldn't talk to me or write me. After I got over there he told me that he was going to divorce me. He couldn't handle it anymore.

I got our unit from Salt Lake City to Fort Carson, Colorado, and then to Germany. After we got there the command in Germany took over. Then I had to get us back home. I knew that this was going to happen. I knew my job was to get us to Germany. When we got to Fort Carson we didn't have an aircraft. So, I had to book an airplane for 245 passengers to take us to Germany. They wouldn't do it at Fort Carson. Our unit was supposed to do it in Salt Lake City and somebody forgot. It was not my job to do it in Salt Lake. We have a command structure in place in Salt Lake. Each portion of that has its specific duties. You have personnel, supply and logistics, the department that is supposed to figure our moving the troops. We had some changes in the unit, and we had a change in the person in charge of logistics.

In Fort Carson I got to pick an aircraft to get us to Germany. I was in this big office with all these people around me and on this computer. They were saying, "We can't touch the computer. You have to put this in here. We'll just show you how." I said, "I don't know how to pick an airplane." I was talking to the Army transportation system online. They, in turn, book an aircraft with Continental Airline. So, I am looking at planes and going, "Okay, this one is pretty. I kind of like the bird on the side of this one. Does it have an engine?" I had all these first-class seats and I wondered what to do with them. I know people are going to be clamoring for these first-class seats. I was very scary to be booking this million dollar airplane. I was scared that we would get to the tarmack and have the wrong sized plane!

Then I had to send this huge MILVAN, probably the size of two banquet tables, to transport all of our duffle bags. A MILVAN is a great big box that goes on a ship. The Army had told us we could take an extra bag. Usually, they only allowed two bags for 18 months. Then they said, "If you want to take a few more things you can put them in this MILVAN." I am booking and signing for this $20,000 MILVAN. This was another thing this person in our unit in Salt Lake was supposed to take care of. Now I own this airplane and this MIL-VAN. I was told that if something happened to this MILVAN while I was responsible for it, I would pay for it out of my pocket. I am responsible for every single thing that went in it. I am responsible if there is anything flammable, so I am inspecting everybody's bag. I am responsible to make sure everything in the MILVAN is going to get there and be sure that nothing is going to have trouble going through customs, which would stop the MILVAN and nobody would get their stuff. I was a one-man TSA. Unit members were mad. They were mad about me inspecting their bags. They were mad because the aircraft could only hold so much weight and only had so much space. Some of the stuff was too big to go over in the plane. I had to explain to them that the aircraft was round and could not take big dresser-sized bags. They had to choose two bags to take over and preferably a duffle bag, which would be round and fit into a round space. I had people yelling at me and it was very, very stressful.

Initially, I wondered why I had volunteered for this position, but I learned a lot. It was a huge job. I had a wonderful mentor, a lieutenant colonel, who has since moved on. He was so smart in everything and so diplomatic. He kind of took me under his wing. He knew I was new to the Army. He knew I had never been enlisted. He knew I didn't even know how to tie my shoe laces. He knew that, but he wanted to help me become a good officer. He never thought any question was stupid. He would drop everything to show me things and to enable me to complete my mission. I could call him at any time and he would answer my questions. He was wonderful and helped me get through the plane and MILVAN thing. He was in Salt Lake City when I was in Colorado by myself, and I e-mailed him a lot.

All the people who were supposed to provide support were in Salt Lake City. You are there all by yourself with all these people that you don't know. Fort Carson deploys soldiers, but they don't do all the ground work. We were there for a month. They provided a place for you to sleep and eat while you are on your way somewhere. They provided a place for us to do our training. We had people from Landstuhl coming to do training about what kind of machines we would be using, all of our HIPAA training. We ran training scenarios, really basic stuff to try and prepare for what we would see in Germany. They were not even close. But it was me trying to figure it out by myself. I was just a little captain, and I have all these people looking at me to get them to Germany. It was very scary.

We finally got everything on the MILVAN and everybody situated on the plane. I dealt with the first-class seats by having a drawing. I knew if I gave the seats to the enlisted, the officers would be upset. I had a full-bird colonel with me. I was afraid she would be mad at me. I just got up there and said, "You know, I know I have a lot of high-ranking officers here. You all probably deserve these first-class seats, but there are a lot of people who have never ever in their whole life had a first-class seat. So what I'm going to do, with your permission and blessing, is raffle off these first-class seats. Just put your name in the hat. We have 15 first-class seats, and we will just draw for them." They all clapped, including the bird colonel. I had a lot of privates who had probably never ever been in a first-class seat who got to fly first class all the way to Germany. It ended up that the colonel pulled a ticket, so she got her seat. But I don't think she would have had a problem with it if she had been sitting in coach. The plane was big enough that there was plenty of space. The Army was very kind to space it all out so that you could have two, maybe three seats in the back. I picked the plane and they told me what my options were. Once we were on the plane, I was very relieved. I figured we were on the plane and out of there.

There were a lot of us over there in Germany with people we didn't know. I was in a room with two women I had never met before. My husband wouldn't talk to me. When we got there we had no sleep. When you first get there they have you drop your bags and show up in the hospital for briefings, two days of briefings with no sleep. Everyone's emotions were kind of high. Then they took you up to the ICU, a very high acuity ICU.

I had a couple of days of orientation in that unit to figure out where everything was. One of the other combat support hospitals was still there and one of their nurses oriented me for two days. It was fast and furious and then that unit left. It was a lot of kind of flying by the seat of your pants. All of the machines you use are different over there. Some of them we were able to touch in Fort Carson, but not everything. The military doesn't have a lot of supplies that other hospitals have. We had the basic stuff.

Everyone thought it would be easier in Germany than in Iraq, but it just wasn't. We weren't on the front lines and we weren't being shot at. I can't imagine being out there being shot at trying to rescue someone or not knowing if where you step you will be blown up. I can't imagine being a medic. My hat goes off to those guys and gals. They are saving people that I'm not sure our best paramedics here could save. We had people who got 40 units of blood before they got to our hospital. How did they get them off the battlefield and keep them from bleeding out and give them that much blood?

Basically, all they did was patch these patients up and send them out to us in Germany. We had patients who had both legs blown off. They would just wash them out a little bit and put some retention sutures in and ship them to us. We got them dirty and bloody with ends of bones hanging out. I had no idea we were going to get them like that. I figured it was an ICU. I knew that we would get people with amputations and gunshot wounds and head injuries. I didn't realize how bad they would look. I didn't realize how labor-intensive it was going to be. One of my goals when I came back was to prepare others for what they would see and prepare them emotionally.

I was not prepared emotionally. My first week I walked into a room and my first patient was 22 and had horrible head injuries. He had been shot through his ear, and it had just kind of gone through his head and sliced his brain in half. He would never be functional again.

One of the hardest things about taking care of this young man was that he looked like my son. He had the same features and the same coloring. His parents had not gotten there yet. I was keeping him alive on vasopressers. I wanted him to look as normal as I could for his parents. I gave him his bath and I would talk to him. I didn't know whether he understood anything or not. I just stood in that room, and he had so many medications going just to keep him alive. His parents got there, and they had not been told anything about the condition of their son. They won't tell them until they get there. They know that they are bad because they won't fly family unless they are pretty bad, if they are severely injured or if there is a question. I don't think they know that they are terminal. They try to keep them alive long enough that their parents can be with them when they die. The parents got there, and the physician took them in and told them what was going on. I was there when the parents came into see their son. I tried to just be part of the wall and just help when they needed help. I tried to let them do what they needed to do. I tried to explain when I was doing something that needed to be done.

The family knew they were going to take him off life support, but they needed to do it when they were ready. They really didn't have a choice. The choice was to harvest his organs or not. However, there was so much red tape getting him back to the states to harvest the organs while he was still alive that it was very difficult to do it for an American citizen. We investigated doing it for a German citizen, but Germany has different criterion for determining death. Portions of his brain were still functioning and the Germans will not harvest in that situation. If he had completely brain dead, they would have taken them. It was hard for these parents because their son wanted to be a donor and there was nothing wrong with his organs. He was healthy and strong.

He had been trached, so when we pulled the tube, he just kept trying to breath. His heart was strong. I was giving the meds and I was trying to help him get more and more sedated as the parents watched this process. The parents were asking me what they should do. I have never had a child die. I've seen people die. I have done the care of the body. I have had grandparents die. But I didn't know what to say to these parents whose child was going to die. I just told them, "Tell him you love him. Tell him it is okay for him to go. Maybe he is hanging on because he doesn't feel like it is okay. Tell him everything you have ever wanted to say because he can probably hear you. Go ahead and touch him, hold his hand, kiss him." He had a little sister, and I asked if she would like to come in. They felt they did not want that, worrying about whether the sister could handle the situation. I am not the one to judge and I would have encouraged them to ask her, but they chose not to do that. They didn't want her in there. It took this man a long time to die. They kept asking me if they were doing the right thing. I had a really hard time with that for a long time. He finally expired and the parents left. I spent the next while wrapping him and getting him ready to be transported.

Soldiers always come across as tough and being able to handle everything, and it is in Germany instead of Iraq so it is no big deal. Boy, it is a big deal. It is bloody and dirty. It is time intensive. It is physical, even more so than in regular hospitals. Because you are lifting and moving off the litters they come on in the transport. They are covered in dirt and there is a bacteria that lives downrange in Iraq. It is called Acinobacter. So, you are completely gowned and gloved to protect you until they come back negative. You can get these bacteria, and you can carry it. If you are a normal healthy adult, it is no big deal. But if you are around someone that is immune-compromised it is bad. It is also something that if it isn't detected can hurt the carrier later. This kind of care is very time intensive.

The patients come in three to fourteen at a time every three days. You are shipping people out every three days. You are getting patients with 90 percent burns. Some of these patients have escharotomies and they are just sliced open. They may be unrecognizable. We are getting these patients to BAMC, Brooke Army Medical Center, the burn center in San Antonio. You don't know if they make it.

Sometimes you will get a patient that you care for over a long period of time. I had one patient that I took care of for 60 to 90 days. I had actually gone down to visit his brother. His legs had been blown to pieces. They were able to salvage his legs, but he got septic from a little piece of shrapnel that had migrated in and perforated his bowel. I didn't think he would make it. I had never seen so many drips on a patient. All I did was run from one machine to another to try and keep the drips going and my drains emptied. It was unbelievable. He eventually left the unit, and sometime later he walked into the ICU and asked for me. He had been getting a little better and then I had been off for three days. While I was gone he had been extubated and moved out of the ICU. We were so busy in the ICU that we didn't have time to go down and visit anybody. He walked in on a day when I was down helping start some IVs in the surgery department. I got my picture taken with him. All the staff came down because they had helped me take care of him.

There was another patient who came walking in after he had left us. He was a young man who was probably 19 or 20. He had drowned. He was in a tank, and his tank turned over in a drainage ditch full of sewer water. He had aspirated and ingested all this sewer water. His lungs just turned to solid masses of crud. He wasn't responsive at all. I didn't think he would make it. You just keep plugging along and trying different things. The Germans have a new machine called a Novalung. It is not FDA approved so we can't use it in the U.S. We shipped this young man to a German hospital and they put on this Novalung. He came walking back in four or five months later. He was on a nasal cannula and will probably always be on one, but he was able to walk back in. We looked at him and said, "You were the deadest dead guy we've ever seen and look at you. You're walking in here." His own lungs recovered. The Novalung is a just a little box that goes in through the femoral vein and the femoral artery and circulates the blood through the box where it gets oxygenated. The idea is to let the lungs recover. It was amazing.

We usually took care of just one patient, sometimes two. It was a lot of work. The patients would come, and you would put them in the room and connect them up to all the equipment. It was all hand charting. There was no computer charting. We usually didn't have anyone to be a clerk. You had to take off all your own orders. We had a couple of people who acted as techs and messengers. You usually had to do everything yourself.

We would float into the short stay surgery department when they got too many patients. The most we got was 26 patients in the short stay, which is a lot when you turn them over every three days. We would stabilize the patients and then fly them out. The Air Force would transport. You packaged them up on their litters, with all their support equipment on a special platform for transport. They went onto a bus and to Ramstein and fly away on a plane. There is one nurse and one doctor on that plane for all the patients who are being transported. The patients have to be pretty stable to be able to fly from Germany to the States.

We had some bomb threats in Germany. We evacuated buildings. We evacuated places at the hospital sometimes. There were certain places we couldn't go if there was any kind of terrorist activities. I was in London the day before the subway stations were bombed. We would get some time off, and they had a really inexpensive mode of travel called Ryan Air. You could fly places for 10 to 25 Euro. That was like $10. They told us to get out of the hospital on our days off, go somewhere, see things, go experience things because it would help your mental status. When I got back to my room from London, all I could do was cry because I had just been there and now I was watching what happened the next day on the news. I just thought, "I was just there. This could have been my friends." So, there were some scares over there.

It was pretty hard being over there, besides the fact that my husband wouldn't talk to me. I had to fly home in June because my brother was having some health issues and my daughter needed back surgery, so I came home to pick a surgeon for my daughter. My husband could have legally done that, but he doesn't have a medical background and would not have felt comfortable making such a decision. They did grant you a certain amount of days of leave. You could take leave to take some time off and you could go anywhere. When you are deployed you can take up to 30 days of leave. They figure it is like a job, and they allow you some reprieve.

After I came back my husband decided he didn't want to divorce me anymore. I don't know what made him change his mind, but he still wasn't very responsive or supportive and he was very angry. At least he was talking to me.

He didn't write me the whole time I was gone. I tried to call him from Germany because it was cheaper for me to call him. I would call every Sunday, but he wouldn't talk to me. We had been married for 19 years. He sent me a card for my birthday and some things for Christmas. I don't know what happened or why he changed. I know it is very, very difficult for a spouse who has never had to be totally responsible for bills, kids, work, yard, housework. I did a lot around our home. He worked hard and was a good provider, but he really never did hands-on with the bills and such. He loved his kids and spent time with them, but he never really did the homework thing and the dinner thing, the woman's work. Plus, we had some rental properties, which I managed. All of a sudden he was saddled with all of this. His comment was, "I have to go to work and then I have to come home and I have laundry and dinner and yard work and kids and rental property, all this stuff." I don't know what happened. Besides, I was playing soldier and he was at home, and I think he has always wanted to be in the military. They wouldn't accept him. He is very much a man's man. Things were tense.

I know a lot of the women over there had similar difficulties. Even some of the women who had an unmarried significant other ended up not having that relationship when they got back. Deployment is very difficult. As a woman, it is very hard to be taken away from your children. You don't realize you can't do anything for them overseas. When your kids are having a crisis, you aren't there. You can't help them when they are depressed or crying or they need their mom. Sometimes only "Mom" works.

I had an episode with my daughter who was having post–partum depression. I was afraid she wasn't going to make it through it. I couldn't go see her and I couldn't leave. On top of that you are dealing with all these soldiers and all their emotions; issues such as lost extremities and females who will never use their hands again, whose faces are burnt, and their anger.

People say, "This war is different than Vietnam. Vietnam was so horrible." Well, I am here to tell you that it is just the same. The soldiers say they never know who is going to blow them up. They can back up five feet and get blown up. They never know if someone is going to walk into their dining room and open fire, even one of their own. People break and they do crazy things. The soldiers are afraid. These women over there are trying to respect the Iraqi people and the Iraqi females. The Iraqi females wanted females to search them. They didn't want males touching them. The American women were there for that reason. They weren't there to shoot at anyone. They were there to help with the border patrols. They got blown up.

When you are over there your comrades are your family. I had more support from those two women that I never met before in my whole life than I had from my husband. My parents were wonderful and they e-mailed me all the time. I had friends who e-mailed me. I had some lady who adopted me in

New Jersey who would send me things. But when it really comes down to the core, those two women I lived with were my family. We talked and cried and we knew all about each other. I don't know what I would have done without them. It is amazing how you create those bonds.

It did give me the same feeling overall that I got when I went to Thailand. I don't know if I would have gotten that same feeling if I had been in Iraq. I don't know that I could have been over there taking someone else's life. As a nurse I was helping our soldiers. I was talking to them. I was comforting them. I got the feeling that I did something good.

People don't understand what is going on or what is happening to our young people. They know how many people die. They don't know how many people are going through the hospital or what their lives are going to be like after they finish. I got a back injury while I was there, but my injury is not even minutely close to what people suffer with. I tried to get into the VA system to have them help me, to let them know that I had an injury in case anything happened in the future. It was like: "We don't have time to see you. We don't want to see you. You weren't shot or burned." I get afraid that all these soldiers will have people turn their backs on them, like the Vietnam era. I find now that we don't have funding for ammunition or training, so I worry about that.

I came back and I felt I had done something good, but I came back with just a little bit of anger about what is happening to all these young people. We have to protect our freedom, but how far are we going to go? How many of these young men and women are we going to continue to send over there to countries that don't want us there and have them blown up? I know there are certain portions of this that we have to do. I am glad to do it. I was proud to serve and I will probably end up going back again, maybe to Iraq.

My unit will probably be mobilized again. Our unit has changed their designation. We are now a rapidly deployable 48 bed hospital for disaster relief. We are the only hospital trained on this equipment right now. There are only six hospitals that have the equipment. It is brand new. I am excited about that. I guess I have a different feeling about war and people inflicting this kind of damage on each other than I do a natural disaster. I feel like with Hurricane Katrina and cleft lips and palates, that people can't do anything about them. They just happen. That is just the way of the world. Helping in that situation would make me sad. People would be injured and maimed. But other people did not cause it.

I had a hard time understanding why I was so angry. I think it is because some of it is so senseless. I feel like the American people are not fully aware of the impact this war is having on not only the soldiers who are coming back with no limbs and unrecognizable, but the impact of sending a soldier over there for 18 months without his family. I think the military needs to rethink some of the things that it does. If you are going to send someone to Germany for 18 months, send the family. Maybe do the deployments in shorter increments, three or six months.

I had a grandbaby born while I was gone that was walking when I came home. I missed all those parts. I missed my girls' first prom. They learned how to drive. I had nothing to prepare some of these soldiers with terrible injuries about how to go on with their lives. I found that the males in our unit had an increased awareness and appreciation for their wives and sweethearts. They had just as hard a time dealing emotionally with being without their kids. It is not a gender issue. It is a separation issue for all the soldiers.

With me in particular, my kids had a really hard time with me being gone. There are certain things that only mothers can do. There are things only dads can do. But men are a little more stoic and have a hard time expressing their emotions and letting others express theirs.

Men were coming home to no wives and were finding out their wives were with someone else. Some of the people in Germany were with people other than their mates. It was the same kind of issues you find in any community and during any war. I don't know if it is people looking for some kind of comfort. I had so many good friends that stood up for what was right and just and who stayed faithful. To me, if you marry someone, you are married to that person. You don't cross that line. It doesn't mean you can't have friends that you talk to. Some of my best friends over there turned out to be men. We would all get together and go on a volksmarch. There are appropriate ways to deal with meeting company and closeness when you are over there without crossing that line. You hate to judge so you kind of keep your mouth shut. There are a lot of people who don't cross the line. They can still talk to the opposite sex. We could all sit down together. We lived in close proximity. We would go to each others' quarters and bring food and we would eat food or have Halloween parties, or we would sit down and watch the movies. You need the companionship. You need to vent and talk about it. You need to be able to talk about what is going on at your house and with your family. It is really hard to keep all that inside.

When I came home my family was doing okay. I only had one brother and he had a significant memory loss due to a traumatic experience while I was gone. I don't know that he will ever recover. So, they had kind of a hard time with that. I had a lot of things happen. Life just goes on without you. But I think they depend on me to do things with him. I go get him and we do things. He has short-term memory loss. He has issues with why they are taking care of a grown man. My parents depend on me to help buffer that. My daughter is doing better now that I am home, but she says, "Mom, there is just nothing like having you home."

I found when I got home that I didn't fit into my family. My husband

and my twins were home and my oldest son was home. He moved out while I was gone and bought his own home and he is doing great. He adjusted well, but he also came over to visit me in Germany while I was there. He came over during Thanksgiving and brought my twins. My husband wouldn't come. I had a hard time fitting back in because they had told us not to go home and start changing things back the way it was. You try to figure out where you fit. They have their own little routines and their own little things, and you find out you don't fit anywhere. The question is, do I start up where I left off before I went away? Do I try to get them back into my routine? Do I leave them the way they were? It was really hard. There was some real tenseness in the family. My husband had a lot of anger still and wouldn't talk to me about it. Subsequently, he left me. I think it was the deployment, but I don't know. It is very, very hard on people. It was an experience I would never trade. I think I helped with the war effort and a lot of it I believe in. Some of it I don't anymore. But it is very hard on families to go through stuff like this. It is the way of the world. War just happens.

The experience was very hard, but the upside to it was that I got to experience a whole different culture. The people that I interacted with living there, the Germans, were so fun. Some of the French were not too friendly. But the Germans were so kind and friendly, kind of "old world," set back in time. I loved that experience. I sort of changed my whole outlook on what was important. Before, I worked three or four jobs, trying to do more and more and more. But I decided I was okay with who I am. Time is too short. You never know when someone is going to take you away from your family. You never know when someone is going to take someone you love away from you, when you are going to lose someone to a war or an accident. It is more important for me to spend time with those people that I care about.

It is more important for me to go back to the basics, to give more of myself as a person, maybe helping someone else through something. I realize how many things someone could be going through. That is why I decided not to do trauma anymore. Not that I wouldn't do it, but I don't want to see the bad parts of life anymore. I want to help somebody be healed or be there for them to talk to me. I work in wound care now. I had a patient the other day that came in and said to me, "I am in here for a wound, but nobody has ever really talked to me like this or really cared about who I am and what is going on with me and why I am sad." Those are the kinds of things I want to do. You don't have to fly half way across the world to do those things. You can do them here. I want to reeducate my children about what is important, the real basics of giving and caring about people. That is what I brought back from that experience with all the things I experienced, as bad as they sound. I think it molded me into a better person.

SUSAN HERRON THOMPSON

Susan Herron Thompson's patient care expertise during her time in the military allowed her to give expert and sensitive service to her patients. Her experience also allowed her to expand herself in nursing expertise and leadership skills far beyond what she anticipated.

My name is Susan Herron Thompson, and I have been in the United States Air Force reserves since December of 1988 when I was commissioned. It was one of those things where I was reading one of my nursing magazines, and it said, "If you want to see the world, join the Air Force." They were right because I've been all over. I knew that I didn't want to spend my weekends in the hospital. That is what I did during the week. The Air Force offered the opportunity to be a flight nurse. I'm a flight nurse. The Army has medevac, which is rotary aircraft, like a helicopter. They'll go in and get them, and then bring them to us. We fly in a large cargo plane, and we do the long haul.

I absolutely think being in the Air Force is part of what I'm supposed to be. I became a nurse by accident. My very first job when I was 16 was in a nursing home, and my job was to wash the wheelchairs, pass ice water, and feed patients. I considered myself an assistant to a nursing assistant. Then I graduated to be a nursing assistant. When I was 18 and graduated from high school and was working at this convalescent hospital full-time, there was a group of people who were going to go down to the city college to take the entrance exams for the LPN program. So I thought, "Hey, I'll go with you." So we went. There were probably six or seven of us that went down. I was the only one that passed. I had to ask myself if I was doing this because everyone else was doing it or because I really want to become a nurse. So I thought, "Well, I'm not doing anything right now." So I went to the LPN program and of course that led to the RN program, which just continued on. I guess for so long I had been working and going to school, doing both at the same time. When I graduated my RN program, I found myself just working for the first time. Then that's when I got interested in the law, so I went to law school and was working and going to school again. When I got finished with that, boom, all of a sudden I'm just working again. I was working at the law firm, and call it boredom or whatever, I guess I just don't know how to not be busy. It was then that I was looking through my nursing magazines and saw the ad and went through the interview and said, "Hey, this sounds great." Now that I'm not working and going to school all the time, I'm working and doing the reserves.

When I joined the military, I think I just became a different person. It caused whatever was in me to sprout and grow. You're forced into different situations; i.e., leadership positions. I hated being put in a leadership position initially. However, once you do it several of times and you start to become comfortable with it, then I realized I kind of like it because now I could set the tone. I could not only do things my way but make sure things ran smoothly and got done efficiently. I think that's the part of the leadership position that I liked, so I knew I was destined for the military. If I had known it was going to be like this, I would have joined years ago.

Going into the military and being in charge of your crew and being responsible and being the coordinator and making sure everything is okay, that's something that really can't be taught. You learn the principles, and then it's up to you to figure out how to apply them.

I remember my mom asking me when I first became a nurse; she said, "Susan, how do you do it? How do you deal with all the stuff you deal with during the day and then come home and be like a normal person?" And I said, "One day as I walked in the hospital and came through the front door, it was like a feeling. I could feel that I became another person." I must have put up that protective wall or whatever it is that you do in order to deal with the patient who has cancer or the child who's dying or the family member that's going through all the grief, whatever it is you do during the day. I think we all have our own protective mechanisms that we put up.

I was deployed three times. I went on Operation Restore Hope. That started in 1992. I was deployed in 1993 for it. It was the famine relief effort in Somalia. You might remember it as Black Hawk Down. It started out being a humanitarian effort. We went there to feed the hungry people, but it didn't turn out like that. I was a flight nurse then, also, and we spent half of our time in Cairo, Egypt, which was where our base was. We would do rotations down into Mogadishu. We spent two weeks in Cairo, two weeks in Mogadishu, two weeks in Cairo, and again two weeks in Mogadishu. Our plane would take off from Cairo, come down, pick up the patients, fly back to Cairo, and then on to Germany. That's where our ultimate destination was to take our patients. If we had a really sick patient who couldn't tolerate a stop in Cairo, we would go all the way onto Germany, which was a ten-hour flight. It was really hard on the patients and the crew. But sometimes you just have to do it.

Operation Restore Hope was a United Nations effort. On the flight line in Somalia, you had the different countries camped all the way around the flight line. There were Americans, Pakistanis, Egyptians, Romanians, Germans and Italians. Every country you could imagine. It turned out really good. If you had some connections, you could go to dinner at a different country every night. We carried a lot of American military, but we also did a lot of humanitarian missions. The Pakistanis got ambushed and there were 50 patients. We regulated those to go to Pakistan, so we actually sent one of our aircrafts into Pakistan. It was the first time in how long? We did not have good relations with Pakistan back then. We sent 50 of their soldiers back with our medical crew taking care of them. That was really cool. We never took any Somalis out. They pretty much stayed in country. I don't remember any of them going out.

There were nurses on the ground as part of the humanitarian mission. The Army was there as the ground unit. They initially were at the flight line as well. They got bombed a couple of times, so they decided it wasn't a good place for the hospital to be. They moved into town, which didn't seem much better. Then they were right in the thick of things. So we would have to convoy initially to go up to the hospital to see patients or to do whatever we needed to do preflight. There are things you got to tell patients or make sure they have before they get on your airplane. Initially we would just get in convoys and go up to the hospital, but pretty soon that became too dangerous because people were getting either sniped or bombed or whatever. So the Army had the helicopters there, Black Hawks, and we would just ride the Black Hawk to the hospital. That was really cool because you don't get to fly in a Black Hawk helicopter all that much. That was a lot of fun. Pretty soon that, too, became very dangerous.

In Somalia it was such a great time, I didn't want to come home. It was an intense experience and I loved it. It's kind of like you leave the stress of your normal life and take on the stress of different life, but this stress is different. It's easier to take initially because it's a different stress. Then this time I didn't really have any preconceived ideas of what it was going to be like because I just had no clue. I knew it was going to be totally different.

When we got there we were separated into crews, so I knew who I was going to be flying with. I had a great crew, people who I flew with all the time at home. Well, I do one mission and then they split the crews up. My second crew was a crew that was at each other constantly, fighting, bickering, and having power struggles. It was horrible. For a month I flew with them on other deployments. I never ever remembered feeling like: "I can't wait to go home." But that's the way I felt during that time. We were on one-year orders with an opportunity to extend for a year, so we didn't know when we were going to go home. I thought, "This is going to last forever and it's going to kill me." Thank goodness at the end of that month the crew I was with was in a special group and they got to go. That was hard, too, seeing other people go home, especially after this difficult time I had been through with this crew. Plus the guy who I had been dating sent me a "Dear John," and it was right at the height of the war. All of these things were hitting me at this one period of time. The next crew, which was my last crew, I spent the most time with, probably two and a half or almost three months with them. They were a great crew, so then I thought, "Maybe I can make it now."

While I was deployed I had been e-mailing a fellow at home. Eventually, he sent me a Dear John." We only started dating two or three months before I left, but it was one of those "talking to each other every day" and "going out every other night" before I left. We were pretty close. I had been gone about two months, and looking back, I can tell that his e-mails had slipped off a little bit. Then I remember the day that I got the e-mail. We would be able to go check our e-mails at either the library or tent or wherever the computers were set up. It was that time when I was on that really hard crew, and when I got the e-mail, it was something I couldn't share with anybody. I didn't feel close enough with anybody on my crew that I could share that or unload that with, so I kept that inside. The other nurse, who was very difficult, was my roommate at the time. After I got the e-mail, I just remember I was walking home in the dark and went in between two buildings where I knew no one would see me, and I just leaned up against the wall and slid down to ground and was just bawling. I had to let it out and that was the only way I could then. That was really hard.

Did I feel like I was threatened? You know it's funny because people ask you that, especially when you get back. They always want to know how close you were to being shot at or something like that. For me, I must always have a false sense of security or I just know that I'm being protected and watched over. Whatever happens is going to happen no matter what. I know I have to be careful, but when you're deployed and you're doing your job, thank goodness I have always felt protected in the back of my mind. I'm not so concerned with safety or something like that. But, we did have a couple of instances.

We had gone in a convoy to the hospital, and there were several of us in the convoy. We were done with whatever we had to do. It was me, one other flight nurse, and the SP. We were in a Humvee and done with our task, so we just thought we would go ahead and drive back. The convoy was still doing their stuff, so they stayed. The Marine that was our SP escort asked if we wanted to take a different way home, because we would always take the same path back and forth. So we're like: "Sure!" We went through a district called K-4. The day after we went through there, we were banned from going through that area because it was so dangerous. We were going down this street and there was a car accident in front of us, so that blocked all the traffic. We didn't know how it happened, but all of a sudden there's like 200 or 300 Somalis coming out into the street. Whenever we drove in a convoy, we always carried a stick because people would reach into your vehicle and try to steal things. As they're reaching in you'd swat them, and that was your protection basically.

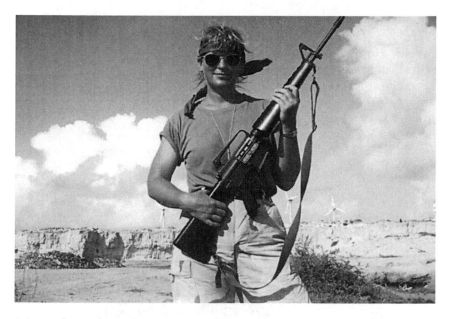

Prior to the conflicts of the late twentieth century, military nurses were not issued firearms. However, Susan Herron Thompson received a weapon for her mission in Somalia and other nurse have reported being issued arms during Desert Storm/Desert Shield and the Iraqi Freedom conflicts.

We all had to carry guns. That was the first time nurses had ever had to carry a gun. You always had your weapon strapped to your chest. On this particular day, the Marine was in the front seat of the Humvee and I and the other flight nurse were in the back seat. This swarm of people started to approach our vehicle, and it wasn't just our vehicle, there were several vehicles. Thank goodness behind us was a UN vehicle with a turret gun. I and the other flight nurse ended up back to back in the vehicle facing our respective window with our sticks because these people were just converging on our vehicle, and they were grabbing at anything that wasn't tied down. Back then they especially wanted your sunglasses. So we're beating people out of the vehicle.

They popped the back of the vehicle and start scrambling in and stealing. It's like you're just beating people right and left. This whole time I kept thinking, "Please don't let me have to pull this gun off my chest and start using it." Then next thing I hear is the nurse who's got her back to me, and she says, "That guy over there has a knife." I kind of looked around and this guy has lifted up his shirt to show that he's got this huge machete stuck down his pants. He was just showing us to let us know that he's got a weapon. The next thing I hear is the Marine, our driver, with his M16 locking up. I'm like: "Oh my goodness, please, please just let us get through here."

I remember thinking at that moment just one of those crazy thoughts that must be like when you think that maybe you're not going to make it back. And my first thought was: "I wish I had a little piece of paper to write a note to my mom and tell her that I love her so I could stick it down my shirt and hopefully somebody would find it." Then I realized, "That's so stupid. My mom knows I love her and I don't need to write a note to tell her." But it's just like I say, it's one of those crazy thoughts that passes through your mind when you don't know what's going to happen next. Anyway, the traffic finally cleared. What seemed like an eternity was probably only about ten minutes. So we get back to the base and I remember that incredible adrenaline surge of thinking, "We made it. That was the weirdest experience and I'm so glad we're here. I will never do it again." But I'm so glad I had that experience because it was so incredible.

I think if you thought about these kinds of experiences and knew that they were going to happen, it would be something that you wouldn't want to go into or do. My mom always used to say that I was looking for adventure, and maybe that's it. But I don't focus on the danger of the experience. I think I always have to ask, "Why am I doing this?" Well, I'm doing this for a reason. "Am I willing to do whatever it takes?" Well, yeah, because I've already made that commitment and taken that oath and that's what's asked of me. Like I say, if you knew it before hand, you probably wouldn't, but you don't know the individual experience that might be the one or the one that comes close. Sure, if we had known that we were going to have our vehicle surrounded and we would have to beat people out of it, we wouldn't have gone that way, but you never know.

Then there was another time. I don't know how threatened we were. I and one of the Army pilots had gotten to be friends. He was going through a hard time at home with his wife and everything. He just needed someone he could talk to. We had concertina wire all around the camp and we were told never to go outside of that. Well, there was this fuel truck with a bench beside it. It was parked just right outside the concertina wire because, of course, you can't maneuver the truck inside of it, so we just walked right outside the concertina wire. We we're just sitting on the bench. You could see the moon and the waves because we were right on the beach. It was a nice place to sit, so we were just talking and chatting. All of a sudden we hear gunfire, and we can see the tracer bullets and they're going right over our camp and right over the fuel truck. So we're like: "Oh, crap." Here it is. It's dark outside. We can't run into camp because camp doesn't know what's going on and all they hear is the gunfire, and if they see people running, they're probably going to shoot us. So we just kind of stayed there waiting to see what was going to happen because there were reports that the Somalis were trying to come over the wall of the camp and invade the camp. So we we're just sitting there and didn't hear anything after that. We waited about half an hour and still nothing, so we thought we needed to do something. We don't know what's going on inside camp either. We figured they might be looking for us. They're probably doing head counts. It was about 45 minutes after the incident. Kind of nice and slowly, we walked into camp talking so they could hear our voice and know that we were coming.

They had black out conditions in the camp, so we made our way to our individual tents. I got into my cot and the person who was sleeping next to me said, "Susan, is that you?" And I said, "Yeah, what happened?" She said that evidently some Somalis tried to come over the fence and the Egyptian guard went crazy and was just shooting randomly all over the place. She said that when the commanding officer came in, she knew who I was with and where I was and that we were chatting right out there, so she said, "I knew where you were, I knew who you were with, so when they came in to do the head count and called your name I just said, 'Here.'" So I said thanks to her. Everything turned out good, but it's times like that that you don't know what's going on. You don't know how threatened you really are. I guess the different countries took turns posting guards on the wall, and he must have seen people coming up. I don't know if he was shooting directly at them or firing warning shots or had too much to drink. Who knows?

When I was young, I always used to think I would die at an early age. Don't ask me why. But that early age I thought was more close to my 20s, and here I am at 43 years old and I'm thinking I haven't had that feeling or thought for a long time. I guess I'm not destined to die at a young age. I had another experience after my mom died. She died in 1997. I had this feeling after she died like: "My mission on earth is complete. I have eased my mother out of this world and have helped to take care of her until she could die. Now I feel like my mission is done." Then I realized I still had my own mission to complete. I guess I just have this innate sense that I'm protected and taken care of and that my Father in heaven is with me. I feel that whatever is going to happen is going to happen, and that's because of the experience that I need to have or the growth I need to make. I don't think everyone experiences this sense. I've had friends in the past who seem to be afraid of everyday life. Part of me, when I sit and listen to them, has a really hard time. "What's the matter with you? That's not right!" And maybe it's the way they were brought up or they didn't have that religious background. To live in fear everyday has got to be hard.

This whole time I was in Somalia I kept thinking, "I can't wait to go home," and I had never felt like that on deployments before. Then I get home and it's like: "I can't wait to go back," because life is so hard now. It's hard to get back into a schedule and routine. I don't know what normal life is like. I don't have a job. Well, I'm still on active duty. I had three weeks off. I was commuting back and forth from Riverside to the base. We get home. We have three weeks off. That was the hardest three weeks of my life. I had people living in my home that were moving out since I was moving back in. I wanted my house back. Then finally I got to live in my house. I woke up every morning and wondered, "What do I do?" There are so many things to do and you're overwhelmed, so you don't do anything. I was finally given the day that I had to start back to going up to the base. It was such a relief and it felt so good to be around people who I had been deployed with, people who had been through the same thing that I had, who understood the stressors. They were all going through the same thing too. It was so good to get back to our family, our military family.

It's weird to be uncomfortable with your own family and to be very comfortable with your military family. That was my life. Now I have more of a level of comfort with my own family. When I first got back, I stayed with my brother for a week because people were still in my house. I didn't feel comfortable there because it wasn't my home. People always want to know how it was and what I did, and if they don't ask, you wonder why they're not. You're uncomfortable sometimes when they do. There are some who say, "I didn't know what to ask or what to say, so I just didn't." You had such a structured life being on active duty for so long, and then all of a sudden there's no structure whatsoever. You felt overwhelmed, so you just didn't do anything because it was easier than having to tackle all these things. I guess for me, I felt like I needed to give myself permission to take a break. I've been through all this, it's okay to just sit on the couch and do nothing. My favorite thing was just flipping through the channels not watching anything because we didn't have TV that we could understand. In Italy, it was all in Italian. In Germany, we did have some TV, but all these places that we'd been, nothing was familiar. The TV shows weren't familiar, nothing. So once I got home, it's like: "I have 96 channels that I can flip through." I wouldn't concentrate on any of them, but just to see what they were.

The three weeks were hard, but I did feel like I needed them, physically, especially because your sleep cycle is weird. It takes time to just get your sleep cycle back on track. When you're deployed, yeah, you slept, but you were always one step ahead of yourself. Alert days were hard because you were always in a state of: "What's going to happen today?" You just never knew.

When I got back, I did not want to share anything. Part of you feels like it's a very personal experience and if somebody hasn't been there, they can't understand it. When they do ask you specifically or they invite you to talk about it, you tend to be very superficial. You tell them pretty much what they already know, what they've seen on the news. Every once in a while you'll interject something like: "The 70 patients…," or something like that. But you never talk about how scared you were when you flew into the desert because of the intelligence briefing you got beforehand, the briefing about how you might get shot and how the RPGs are located and what they're aiming at, about the chemical possibilities and how you're having to strap on all your chem. gear when you land in the desert. The first several weeks when we flew in, we were getting these intelligence briefings, and that was enough to scare the crap out of us. So that was hard. You don't talk a lot about that stuff.

Unfortunately, it wasn't 'till about three or four months after we got back that our squadron had a debriefer. We didn't get debriefed 'till everybody's pretty much getting over it. And we had already talked amongst ourselves.

We went through about a month where everybody in our squadron didn't really say anything until one person said, "Are you having any difficulties now that we're back?" And I said, "Yeah!" Then a couple other people, we asked them, and it turns out that everybody is having some sense of difficulty. Maybe not the same, but in some facet of their life they're having some difficulty. Especially the ones in my squadron that were deployed at the same time, I still keep in touch with them. I see them every month. That's very nice because we all have a bond. The other people, we have bonds with them, too, but it's a little different, it's not as strong. There are a couple other people from different squadrons that I ended up flying with that I still keep in touch with. That's really neat to see what they're going through now. I got an e-mail from one of the guys I flew with the longest, best crew, and he talked about some of the difficulties he'd been through, so I wrote him back. He wrote me back and said, "I don't know if you knew this, but every time something happened or something came up that was difficult on the mission, I always kind of turned to you for validation or to make sure it was okay or what I did was right." I thought that was so sweet. I never realized that. But it's nice to hear stuff like that, especially with him because I looked at him being the guy in charge. He was the strong man, but never showed his fear. That's the sign of a good leader is not showing how scared you really are.

We knew that Iraqi Freedom was coming up, but we didn't know when. They were asking for volunteer lists because we have a squadron of 150 people. In an air evac squadron, they usually don't deploy your whole squadron. They usually take bits and pieces and make their own squadron with a bunch of different people. So when we knew that the war was coming up, boy, I was like: "Are you sure I'm on the volunteer list? I want to see it." Then when we got the call, it was like: "Uh oh. This is really going to happen now." But I knew that because I have over 15 years in that this might be my last chance for a war and my last chance to do what I've been trained to do. Maybe you get psyched up your whole career because this is what you're trained to do and then finally you're able to do it. There are several people in our squadron like me. Then there are several people like: "Hey you know what, I joined to go to school and to get benefits and I've got a family now." I totally understand that. I can't even imagine being a regular reservist and having children and being gone one weekend a month let alone to be deployed away from your home when you have kids. So I'm so thankful that my life worked out to where I've been single and I can just float around and go wherever I'm asked to go. But I remember thinking, "This might be my last chance for war, so I'll go."

Each deployment is different. For Desert Storm, I was in England. It was a party time. We never saw a patient. We never got on an airplane, never flew. Restore Hope was half party, half scary. Half of it was a really great time. When we were in Cairo, we were in five star hotels and catered to. It was just wonderful. Then when we were in Somalia, we were in a tent in the middle of a desert, but still that was great. During Iraqi Freedom it was totally different because there was no fun and game time. There was none of that party time or that let down and relax time. In those seven months, I would venture to say I had five days off. On those five days, if you were in England, you went down into London and that was your day off. Once we were in Sicily, we went to Mount Etna. Two more times I had days off in Germany and that was pretty much it. Your other days were spent getting ready for the mission, doing the mission, or recovering from the mission. Then you started up that whole cycle again. I don't think of myself as being an adventurer. I think of myself as having a pretty mundane life that every once in a while has these blips on the screen of excitement. When I was deployed for Desert Storm, we were only gone for three months, so that wasn't a big issue. We didn't see anything there. We heard on the news, but CNN was as close as we got to the war.

For Iraqi Freedom we had a very complicated thing to start with. My group was initially sent to England. We started out in England, and then we would fly down to Sicily. We would sit alert in Sicily, then we would go from Sicily to Kuwait and pick the patients up, and then fly them to either Germany or Spain. It was a big huge circle. As the war progressed, they eliminated some of these spots. Pretty soon we ended up going from Germany to the desert, Germany to the desert, etc.

The planes that we flew usually were the C-141s. They have the capability of transporting 103 litter patients, and then a mixture if you have ambulatory patients. We had a combination of patients. Some of the patients would come on the plane with only a diagnosis of an abnormal pap smear. Other patients would come to us on ventilators with head injuries or blast wounds or burns. You saw everything. In Germany we had Landstuhl, a big hospital there. It had the capability for everything. It could handle trauma and all kinds of stuff.

After we took care of the service members, we never really knew what happened to them. What we did know is that we took them to Germany, and then occasionally we would do a mission to the United States, and we would bring some of the more serious ones stateside. We never really saw them after that. I'm assuming there were many that returned to duty.

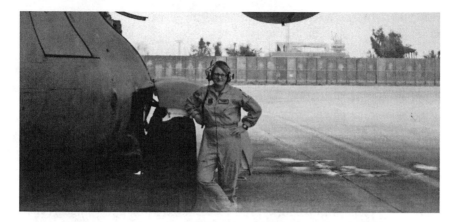

Most of the time Susan Herron Thompson flew in a C-141. It could transport 103 litter patients and a mixture of ambulatory patients.

We were deployed from February 2003 and we returned stateside in August, so about six to seven months. We seemed to never stay in one place for more than two days. We were in England for two days, then we would fly to Sicily, then we would crew rest, get ready for a mission, and stay there for two days, and then go to Kuwait. At the initial part of the war, we would just land in Kuwait and go on, and that made a 24-hour workday for us. We would be dead after that. Then they decided that they were killing the air evac crews, so they decided to allow for crew rest. Even then, when you hit Kuwait you had to off load all the cargo that they put on your plane, and set up everything for your air evacuation. By that time, you were 12 hours into your day and you're dead tired already. It's also 120 degrees outside, and you're in a hollow metal tube.

You would pick up all your patients, and then fly to Germany. That was another overwhelming thing. When we were in Sicily, we would get a basic initial report of how many patients we were going to get. They would tell us that we would get 20–30 patients, and that in itself was kind of overwhelming because you have three nurses on the plane. So then you land in Kuwait and they come on the plane and say, "Oh, you're getting 70 patients today." Seventy patients! It was crazy.

Our patients were mostly active duty. We did have a couple of Iraqi nationals. Most of them were humanitarians. I remember one was a 16-year-old girl who had burns. Another one was an Iraqi freedom fighter. There were a couple others interspersed in there. Most of the time they had an interpreter with them. That really helped. Otherwise, it's body language. Especially if you're dealing with the males, you have to be very careful because having a female touch them or even approach them is something you just don't do. You really had to keep that in mind. Americans are very touchy-feely. That's how nursing is.

There were three nurses on the flight crew. One nurse would be the medical crew director who was in charge of paper work and coordination and all that kind of stuff. The other two nurses would split the plane in half. One nurse would take one side of the plane and the other nurse would take the other side of the plane. So you started at one end of the plane, and you just worked your way down. You gave your medicines and did your bandaging, started your IVs, gave your morphine pushes, charted when you could, and did whatever you had to do. By the time you finished and got down one side of the plane, you had to start all over again.

We have very strict guidelines and regulations on narcotics. When a client comes on a plane with narcotics, you do a double count and you chart that. When you have 70 patients and at least half of those are coming on with orders for tons of morphine, there's no way to count it and there's no way to account for it. You're just pushing morphine and hopefully being able to chart on it because you've got so many morphine pushes to do. Everything takes so much time, such as being careful about mixing your drugs. We were mixing all of our IV antibiotics since nothing came premixed. It was very overwhelming.

One of the things I realized when I got back into the urgent care emergency room at the VA was that there were some days that I really enjoyed my job and other days where I felt this stressful feeling. I realized that I was having some.... I don't want to call them flashbacks because that just sounds so veteranish, but it was that overwhelming feeling, the feeling of being overwhelmed and being out of control and not knowing if you could do it because there are so many things that needed to be done. Like when we have 50 patients out in our waiting area, they all need to be seen now, and you can't get to them all. It's just like 70 patients being on your plane and each one of them needs something, but you can't do everything. Again, it was that overwhelming feeling that I felt during the war, and I didn't like that. I started to think that it was time to go on to a more structured environment, so I started looking for another job position.

Sometimes training for war is different than going to war. They tell you to train the way you're going to go to war, so we train a certain way. We have our medical supplies packaged a certain way. We go on training missions. During our weekend training missions we're going to bring on our supplies and we're going to set up the plane. We will have people playing patients and people playing crew members. We will have diagnoses for these patients, and we will have to go get supplies out of our kits to take care of these patients. That's how we train. Well, I don't know when it was, whether it was the week we left before the war or the week after we got to the war, but they changed the packaging guidelines. The theory was if you have between 10–20 patients, you're going to take bags #1–3, so you only have to take three bags. If you have patients 20–30 or 20–50, you're going to take two extra bags. Now that's five to seven bags we're up to, and it was still manageable. If you have fewer patients, you'll take fewer bags. However, like I said, in Sicily we were told we were going to have 20–30 patients. By the time we get to Kuwait we're told we have 70 patients. We ended up bringing every single piece of equipment and every package of bags full of all our stuff on each and every mission. Now that the packaging guidelines are different, we don't know where to go, which bag is what. The new guidelines didn't really help because we had to take everything anyway. When you're looking for IV tubing, which used to be in bag # 3, but you'd have to look through the packaging guidelines, 16 pages of the packaging guidelines, to figure out which bag it was in, and your patients are screaming in pain.

You don't have time to be looking for stuff like that. It was very frustrating to have things change right before we went to the war. Initially, we had enough stuff because we were only carrying 20–30 patients during the first couple of weeks of war. After that is when we started getting our missions of 50, 60, 70, and sometimes up to 80 patients. Then we started running out of things like saline flushes, piggy backs, tubing, needles, syringes, or other things you were using all the time for a lot of patients. What we as individual flight nurses started doing after every mission was to repack our kits. We all had our own little kits, our own personal bags that we would throw in a bunch of extra stuff, the stuff we knew we were going to be using a lot. We all had extra supplies with us. Not being prepared happens to you once and you learn. Then the rest of the time you're prepared.

On our airplane we had three flight nurses and four medical technicians on every flight. Many times we would have a CCAT (critical care air transport) team. That consisted of a doctor, a critical care nurse, and a respiratory therapist. They would take no more than three patients. They could take three critical patients, but no more than that. We would give them our three worst patients and we would do the rest. That was usually the ventilator and the cardiac monitor guy and somebody else who required suctioning or stuff that required hands-on every so often. The form has a patient's name, their diagnosis, doctor's orders and a place for nurse's charting. You would look at that. Half of the time it's old because they've been in the system for at least 24–48 hours. You're looking at these old orders. Sometimes you'd have patients puking their guts out because they're air sick, but you have no orders for Compazine or Phenergan or anything. Those were the times that we were thankful for the CCAT doc to write an order. We do have a couple standing orders. Sometimes the doctors would be good about writing standing orders or PRNs, but if they did not, in our regulations we have certain drugs that we can give as one time doses. Nothing push or nothing IM, it's all PO. Well if they're vomiting, they're not going to be able to keep POs down. You just do what you can and hope you don't run out of barf bags.

I got to the point where I would carry around Dramamine everywhere because I never get airsick except on these missions. That was probably because of the length of the day that once that fatigue hits, you're just susceptible to everything. I remember two missions specifically where there was something wrong with the autopilot, and we were listing the whole time and everyone was throwing up. We were pushing Phenergan like crazy. The crew members would go in the corners and throw up in the barf bags and then go about their duties, then go and throw up again. We had no pharmacy support. For the really sick patients, we'd get either a bag or a box with all their medicines. You made sure during training missions that you had the right supplies requested. But during the war you hoped you had what you needed and you just made do.

I would say during the height of the war, we did a lot of putting out fires because you came up on situations that you hadn't encountered before that you can't anticipate, so you were reacting. As we learned the kinds of things that were happening, we knew that we were still going to be facing a lot of this stuff. You learn to be more prepared and to be able to act. After every mission, our entire crew would get together and we would debrief. We would actually have to do a written debrief for our commander about the problems we encountered and the solutions we implemented and the things we wanted to have change. We would give as many suggestions as possible.

We got along well with the other services. We worked a lot with the Army. The Navy, I don't think we had a whole lot of interaction with them other than as patients. They mostly got flown out on a helicopter and put on the boat because the boat was right off the land there. We had lots of patients from the Marines, especially 18- or 19-year-old kids. That was hard. There were kids with now no arms, legs, or eyes. I remember one kid that was sitting next to me. He came on the plane and took off his helmet. So he takes of his helmet and is looking at the inside and I glanced over to see that he had a picture of his little baby girl with his wife. That was enough to break my heart. He turned to me and said, "I just missed her first birthday." That was hard because all of a sudden they became human. They became real. They weren't just patients. They weren't just the belly wound or the burn. They were people and they had families and they were just like us.

You try to always have a smile on your face. You always greet them. You always talk to them. They had been eating MREs forever, months and months. So, the crew would take up a collection and we would all donate between five and ten dollars. This particular mission, we would do once a week. We would donate money and go to the commissary and buy hot dogs, cookies, and French fries. We had these little ovens on the plane. We would cook hot dogs, cookies,

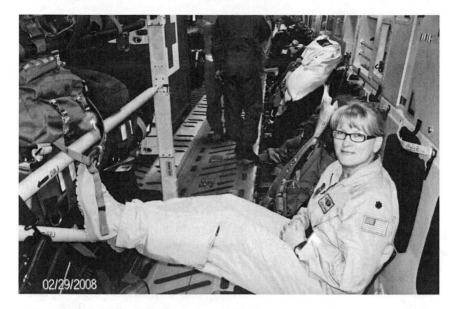

Even though this plane could hold a lot of patients, either on a litter or standing, space was at a minimum. Susan Herron Thompson in 2008.

and French fries. These guys must have thought they had died and gone to heaven because they had not had real food in so long. It was the coolest thing.

We had a fireman on our crew for most of my flights. Somebody sent him this huge American flag and we would hang it inside the aircraft. When the patients saw this, they knew they were going to get some food. You always had to think of their morale, because we always knew that they had been through the worst of it. It wasn't us. We still got to stay in a bed and shower and go eat at restaurants. We had those things, but they didn't.

In the beginning, when they came on the plane, you could tell they had been through something because of their affect and their look on their face. You could smile and do whatever, but they wouldn't respond as much. Some would, but some wouldn't. Then they all seemed to be in a phase where they were much happier and much less stressed. Then I remember when we started doing the mission straight into Iraq.

What would happen was we would pick up the patients in Kuwait. They had a 130-unit plane, a smaller plane. They would go to Baghdad and Tikrit and Kirkuk and bring the patients down to Kuwait where we would pick them up. Well, we started doing missions directly into Iraq and into Baghdad and bringing them straight to Germany. This was probably after the major fighting had gone on and I was ground supporting Germany. We recovered this plane that had just come in from Baghdad. These people had the flat affect and no energy and they were quiet. It was weird to see that again. You knew that they had been through some stuff. It's hard because you can't talk on the plane. You can't hear. You have earplugs in, the plane is so noisy, and you have to yell even at a close distance. Sometimes you could carry on conversations on the rare occasion that you had a lull in what you were doing because you had an eight-hour flight. The techs were able to chat more because they had fewer duties than the nurses. I would see the techs going up and down the aisle talking to people. Most of the time, the patients just slept. They were exhausted

I would do it again. Maybe that's a personal thing, but yeah, in a heartbeat I would do it again. Had you asked me if I would do it again right when I came back ... see when we got back, they were asking for volunteers who wanted to stay on active duty and probably go out again soon, and I said no to that. I was dead when I got back — mentally, physically, psychologically, spiritually, and emotionally. I felt like my sense of joy had been taken away, and it was so hard to integrate back into normal life, back into my family life, back into my home life, my friends. It was so hard. I don't remember it being that hard before with other deployments or coming home from my mission or other stretches of time of being gone. So, right when I came back, I said I was never going anywhere again. But here, I've recovered and am back to normal life, and, oh, yeah, I would go back again.

Through church, I had a real great support. That was really nice. I would get a lot of e-mails. Every week the achievement day girls would get together and spend the last five minutes of their meeting writing to me. Their leader would then send all their cards to me. That was really special. Every week I would get a packet.

I have two big brothers, neither one has been in the military. My dad was actually in the Navy for four years during Korea. They didn't call them this back then, but he was a SEAL. He was involved in underwater demolitions and all that good stuff. UDT is what they called them then. It's funny, because once I joined the military, he started opening up and telling me a couple of stories. Then when I would go on deployments, especially after Somalia because I would write back all the time, he would open up a lot more, especially now, after this one. I got back in August. My dad was a fireman, and he got emphysema really bad because he was a smoker, plus all the smoke from the fires, so he just moved in with me in November. He lives with me now and we have more opportunity to talk. It's nice to talk about things with my dad, especially about things that he's kept in for so many years.

He worries a lot, especially now. When he was living in Georgia, he didn't know when I would go off on the weekends or whatever, but now that he's living with me, he knows. This weekend I'm going to be gone on a three-day mission, and he worries now because our planes are old and they're falling apart. He would never tell me how much he worried, but when I got home and some of the things he said, I could tell that he was definitely worried. But he didn't want to let on to that because he wanted to support me. He didn't want me to worry about him worrying. He was very supportive and wrote me a lot. Most of the time when I received his letters, it was great. He had a very difficult living situation back home. His wife is an alcoholic. That's one of the reasons he lives with me now because life back there got so dangerous. He would write me about how he almost ended up in the hospital or how he did go to the hospital because he couldn't breathe. He had to call a cab because his wife was too drunk to take him. I was like: "There's no one taking care of him!" But thank goodness his church was there and they were looking after him. It was hard getting the bad news because being the daughter, I'm the caretaker of the family. When something happens, that's my job. Being that far away, you have to just trust the rest of your family. I would write my brothers and tell them they need to call Dad once a week without failing. For the most part, it's good to hear from home. After a while, it's like: "I hope no one else writes me because I don't feel like writing back." I just felt obligated if someone wrote to me to write back, but that got so hard. To a certain extent, I wanted to forget about life back home. When I first left, and maybe this was one of the reasons I got a "Dear John," I did not call him. I would e-mail him, but I did not call him. I needed to make a break with home, and the way I did it was no phone calls. I e-mailed everybody but I didn't maintain telephone contact. So you do need to break it off to a certain extent. I didn't want to know if my cat had to go the vet. I didn't want to know if my plumbing broke. But I'd still hear about all this stuff and it got to be hard, so I would tell my brother to just take care of things.

We have rotations right now. There's one going out in March. There are enough volunteers for that. There's another one going out in June sometime. I haven't heard if they have enough volunteers for that or not. Now normally I would say that I would go in June, but right now, now that my dad just moved in with me, I'm kind of in a different living situation with different responsibilities, so I have to think more about what I need to do versus what I would like to do. Right when I first started back here in my job, I wanted to go back because it was hard being integrated back into work again. But now I'm getting used to that.

Who knows now at this point when I'll go. I'm kind of waiting for my dad to stabilize with his emphysema. If it was just selfish me, then I would go with the next wave. It's a responsibility issue now. I have two brothers, but guys just don't see things the same way. Maybe guy nurses are different, but my brothers ... we'll be all in the same room and none of them would see how my dad was suffering with his breathing. My brothers are more unifocal, whereas women, we can be doing something but we know what's going on other places.

The Association of Military Surgeons of the United States has a conference every November, and I was fortunate enough to be one of the presenters. There were like 5,000 people there. Now the time I presented, there were probably only 200 because it was one of the breakout sessions. But one of the speakers talked about how he had just gotten back from Iraq and how misleading the news is. All we see is how all these Americans are being killed and shot and all the money we're spending and how the Iraqis are still shooting at us and hating us. He said, "When we go to Iraq, when they see an American, they run up and hug us and thank us and they are so grateful to us. They now have clean water, they now have food to eat, and they now have medical systems. They now have an infrastructure." He's talking about how all these people are so grateful for the things that they have now and the change that has happened. I think now's the time when they need to have the reporters embedded in these units so they can see what's really going on and the good that we're doing instead of getting the negative aspect from the news. So every chance and every opportunity I get, I tell people about that.

JANE VALENTINE

Jane knew she wanted to do something special, so she became a nurse, made the decision to join the Air Force Nurse Corps and then to become a flight nurse. Those decisions placed her in a position to make a difference in the lives of many colleagues and patients. Some of Jane's Air Force experience prior to her assignment in the Persian Gulf has been included as it has bearing on her activities while in the Persian Gulf.

Scott Air Force Base (AFB) had one of the few aeromedical evacuation squadrons (AES) in the Air Force. Additional squadrons were located at Travis AFB, California, the Philippines, and in Germany. I thoroughly enjoyed my job at the Scott Medical Center, but as I passed my two and a half years on station, I sought the opportunity to attend Air Force flight nurse training and wanted to obtain a flying assignment overseas. Flight nursing was highly competitive with many wanting a chance at the limited slots. I was focused on my job at the medical center, but keep an eye on my dream to become a flight nurse. One day I received a call to report to the Military Airlift Command (MAC) Surgeon General's office which was located at Scott AFB. The command surgeon general stated he had heard of my interest to be a flight nurse and knew it may be a big driver in my interest to continue my Air Force career. I expressed my commitment to the Air Force but certainly being a flight nurse was my career goal. Pilot training was not yet being offered to women in the Air Force and this offered an avenue to learn more about the line of the Air Force and its flying mission. Flight nursing also offered a unique opportunity to practice nursing in an arena that could not be matched in the civilian sector. The next thing I knew, I was on my way to flight school at Brooke Air Force Base in San Antonio, Texas, for training. I was notified while in flight school that I would be given a flying assignment for my next assignment. Shortly upon my return to Scott AFB, I was notified of my assignment to Rhein-Mein, Germany, at the 2nd Aeromedical Evacuation Squadron. I knew then that what started as a two-year Air Force assignment, now extended at least three more years and most probably an Air Force career.

My flight assignment at Rhein-Mein was three years, September 1979 through August 1982. Once again, I had a lot to learn and every mission offered new exciting adventures. I was tri-qualified in three aircraft; DC-9s, C-141s and C-130s. Our squadron flew missions within the European theater (usually DC-9s) and twice weekly there were stateside missions (C-141s) to Andrews AFB, Maryland. The 2nd AES supported transporting injured U.S. troops and dependent family members stationed throughout Europe to larger U.S. medical facilities in Germany and stateside if needed. As a flight nurse I flew all over Europe, with an occasional overnight stay in Ankara, Turkey. That was an interesting experience. Billets were bare-boned, and sometimes we only had large trashcans filled with water to wash up. One of the most significant events while in Germany, was meeting my future husband, Russ, a C-130 pilot and flight examiner, soon after my arrival on base.

While 2nd AES flew routine routes weekly, there was a need to send alert crews on urgent missions as acute medical emergencies arose. When on alert crew status, I never knew when there would be an urgent mission and what it would entail. I was involved in two very significant and, in fact, historic events. One was April 1980: I was sent, in the middle of the night, to a secret location to air evac those injured in a hostage rescue attempt. This was especially harrowing, as we were briefed that a C-130 aircraft was involved and Russ had also been deployed earlier to an unknown location. I was relieved when I was informed that the 37th TAS (Russ's squadron) was not involved in the crash. But both Russ and I were shocked to see each other on the desert tarmac as both were alerted to the same location. Another significant alert mission involved evacuation of injured from the October 1981 assassination of Egyptian President Anwar Sadat. This experience in working closely with the line of the Air Force made this assignment one of my best.

Before leaving Germany, Russ and I got married and we worked a joint spouse assignment. Russ already had orders to a staff job at the MAC headquarters at Scott Air Force Base, Illinois. I was told that a move back to Scott AFB for my overseas follow-on assignment could be detrimental to my career, as I had already had an assignment previously at that location. Of course, I chose to take my chances and requested an assignment to Scott AFB. I certainly did not want to be separated from my new husband. Despite this move, I was selected for promotion to the rank of major two years below the zone; therefore, I clearly overcame the risk of this negatively impacting my career. This was quite a busy assignment for me — a new husband, instant family (Russ had two children, Melanie and Adam), a promotion to major and new baby girl, Ashley.

I stayed at Scott AFB for over four years and had successive promotions. I was first the infection control officer (August 1982 to July of 1984); then charge nurse surgical unit (July 1984 to June 1986); and coordinator, outpatient nursing services (July 86 to July 87). When the Air Force developed their new ambulatory service model, I became the director of ambulatory services (DAS), which aligned nursing, medical staff, and ancillary services under this position (April 1987 to Sept 1988). This position certainly was a challenge, but through careful collaboration, we were very successful.

At this time I was due for a new assignment, and once again Russ and I looked for a joint spouse opportunity. The best we could find was for me to go to Seymour Johnson Air Force Base while he went to Pope Air Force Base. Russ's assignment opened up first, and he departed for North Carolina with Adam while I stayed at Scott Air Force Base. (Melanie was living with Russ' ex-wife in Germany.) We sold our house, and I became virtually a single parent as Ashley and I moved into a townhouse together. About 18 months later I finally got my orders for Seymour Johnson AFB, NC, and joined Russ and Adam.

Our two bases, Seymour Johnson AFB and Pope AFB, were too far apart to live at one of them. We moved between the two locations to Four Oaks, North Carolina. Four Oaks is a small rural town with very little connection with either military base. Russ went west to work and I went southeast. But this at least kept us living in the same household. Seymour Johnson was my first chief nurse position, and I had long looked forward to this position. I had excellent mentors over the years that provided advice, guidance, and through their high expectations for performance, taught me much about nursing leadership. Colonel (retired) Nancy Caldwell was especially an outstanding role model — she was tough, but I contribute much of my success today due to her mentorship. I felt more than ready for this position. I was excited about this challenge; and our joint spouse arrangement worked fairly well until my deployment to the Persian Gulf War.

I arrived at Seymour Johnson October 1988 and was promoted to lieutenant colonel February 1989. Contingency planning and the possibility of deployment were well understood. The 4th Medical Group's mission included supporting a prepositioned air transportable hospital (ATH) somewhere overseas. We trained for this contingency throughout the year. Many AF bases actually had their ATH located on base with them, and in fact, they trained regularly with their own equipment and supplies. However, at Seymour Johnson we trained with what materials were provided; not as ideal as having our actually ATH, but effective. Deployment training was as much a part of life in the Air Force as direct patient care. It was continuous and a priority. It caused unique staffing challenges, as we had to support mobility lines and simulated deployment on base throughout the year. It was August 1989 when our hospital executive team was notified that we were deploying in support of Desert Shield. We had approximately a week's notice to have our personnel ready.

We made the deployment announcement to our staff, and there were a lot of mixed emotions. While our staff had been training for the possibility of deployment all along, now they would be applying that training in reality. A lot of the staff were very young, in their 20s, and were excited about this expe-

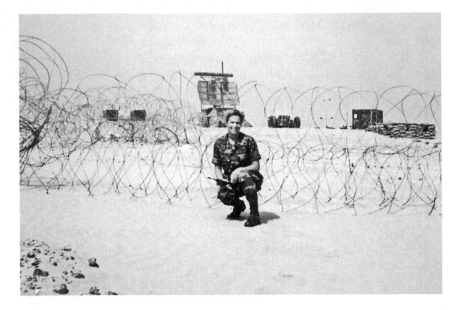

Jane Valentine with the base in the background. Security was paramount, which included the base perimeters protected by surveillance, natural berms, and razor wire.

rience. They were all very patriotic and were proud to be called upon to deploy. They were ready to go. I was also very proud of all of them — and their families who supported them. We had a number of dual married Air Force couples, where both individuals were scheduled to deploy. While all of us in the military are obligated to make personal arrangements for our children in case of deployment, we were able to offer one of each of these couples the option to remain stateside, as we had individuals who volunteered to take their deployed position. But not one stayed behind. In all cases, both were both committed to the mission and determined to go.

Despite the deployment of nearly two thirds of our hospital staff, I was still expected to retain operations. I relied on middle managers to move into higher leadership roles until the reservists were deployed to backfill our hospital. We were informed that three of our manifested positions would be filled by Air Force medical readiness staff from another base to assist our team with setting up the air transportable hospital once we were at our deployed location. One of the executive leadership team had to stay behind. I gave up my position to work the details on how the Seymour Johnson Hospital would maintain its support to our base personnel and patients. The amount of the delay was not known but estimated to be days to perhaps a week.

One of my first major concerns was how to provide emergency response support to the base with the majority of my emergency room staff deployed.

Fortunately, I was able to pull together sufficient qualified emergency room nursing and technician staff. However, I identified the possible risk in on-base response secondary to delays from the unfamiliarity with finding locations in a timely manner on the base. Staff were deployed that quick — here today and then flying out within weeks. Therefore, until the staff was proficient in locating the calls, we utilized our base security police to provide police escort for emergency calls.

One item that made this deployment unique for me was the fact that our deployed location was classified. The Air Force had pre–positioned ATHs and hospital equipment supplies in warehouses all over the world depending on where it was thought a contingency would develop. We had no idea where these were stored. We only knew we were going to be connected to one in theater.

There were 130 people from our hospital that were slotted to deploy in support of the air transportable hospital (ATH). I cannot recall exactly how many we had assigned at our hospital at that time, but this deployment took probably a good two thirds of our personnel. We had multiple reserve units that trained with us and hoped that they would backfill our staff if deployment occurred. It seemed logical since these reservists were fairly close by and it was more cost effective to train locally. I had planned on this pool of experienced reservists that were very familiar with our hospital operations, as they trained side by side with us. In fact, I had several Nurse Corps officers that would train with me in the chief nursing position. However, the contingency plan did not place these reservists at their training locations. Instead, I found that many were deployed across the U.S. Unfortunately, the reservists that came to fill our vacancies had never been there before. But Air Force hospitals are fairly standardized in their operations, and we had structured policies and continuity mechanisms in place to ensure their success. Air force personnel, active duty or reservists, are very resilient and have the ability to take available resources and make it all work. They did that and the stateside mission was executed superbly.

After a couple of weeks, I was notified to join our 4th Medical Group contingent. We had gotten word back that our hospital commander developed kidney stones and was returning back to Seymour Johnson for medical care. This was at the moment when I was deploying to join the 4th Medical Group. This would be good for the 4th Medical Group in North Carolina, but I wondered about the leadership of the ATH at the still secret deployed site.

When my deployment orders were cut, I realized that we were sent over in troop components that consisted of approximately twenty-five personnel. A lieutenant colonel at the time, I was the senior ranking officer and therefore designated as the troop commander. My troop was not a medical deployment contingent but a collection of personnel that needed to get over to the European theater to Rhein-Mein, Germany, where they would receive their next orders. When we departed we did not fly straight to Rhein-Mein, but actually took five days, which included two stops. The first was Dover Air Force Base where we stayed for two nights. There were not any billets set up for those traveling; that was left up to the troop commander to establish once I arrived at each location with the base personnel. I had full responsibility to care for those traveling in my troop. I knew basic needs of shelter and food were critical. At Dover AFB I was only able to find some space in a base recreation center, as we were not allowed to use off-base billets. We had cots and set them up with the males located on recreation main floor and the women on the stage. This provided some privacy. We were supplied basic sleeping materials such as blankets, and we had our personal mobility bag. Our second stop was a short layover in Loring, Maine, before arriving at Rhein-Mein, Germany.

When we landed at Rhein-Mein it was crowded, and it suddenly became clear as to the magnitude of this massive deployment. The reality of the pending war also began to set in with the deployed troops. We had six or eight hours before we left again, and I was told to have my new troop component ready to go. The base had cookies and sodas for those waiting, and I was told to have my troop contingent all back at a central location at a certain time. I was not told that I had to have my troops remain there at all times. Having been stationed at Rhein-Mein, I was familiar with the facilities. I thought that perhaps some of these personnel may not even return from this conflict. Maybe it was a little dramatic, but I thought, "I'm not going to make these guys hang around in this hanger eating cookies with the local wives' club if they are about to deployed to the desert." I picked out the most senior NCOs in the group and told them that I would hold them responsible to get them back in time if they preferred not to spend the time in the combined enlisted-NCO Club. They could not have been happier; and all showed up on time.

From Germany we hopped on a plane and went to Saudi Arabia, landing at Dhahran, which was the central hub for Air Force deployed troops. We had masses of people moving through this area, and the infrastructure was not yet established to accommodate all of the people. We loaded on a bus and were told, "We are going to take you to a warehouse. You may want to tell your people to grab some cardboard, if there are any cardboard boxes, because that may very well be what you will be sleeping on." While speaking with a forklift operator in the warehouse, I told him I was going to wherever the 4th Medical Group was located. He said, "Oh, down there in Oman." So my medical group's contingent secret location was known by a forklift operator and finally by me. I was relieved to at least know of a location.

My number one priority was to make sure my troop component was fed and had a decent place to sleep — we were not sleeping in the warehouse on cardboard. It was noisy, dirty, dusty and hot! I grabbed one of my senior NCOs, and we set out to find a place that was at least air-conditioned. We were offered a school, but we would have to sleep in a hallway where we would not be able to turn off the lights. This was also located a bit of a distance from the base. That would definitely not work, but it was shelter (better than cardboard on a warehouse floor). We then found a building that had an available room with pool tables, nearer the base, with a bathroom down the hall and access to where food was provided. We had one couch in this room, but no one would take the couch. I had to practically force someone to sleep on the couch. Others slept where they could find space, under the pool table or on top of the pool table. It was air-conditioned and was functional. We found a place to wash up, get fed and grabbed our new-found space.

As the troop commander through this part of the journey, I met with a number of personnel officers. They had their hands full, trying to keep the troops moving out, only to have more waiting to come in. It was amazing how it all worked, despite the constant input of more troops. My troops were sent on their way, and I waited for my own final departure for Thumrait, Oman, to meet up with the 4th Medical Group hospital contingent. I waited for my flight call in a holding tent right off the flight line. While these were not very comfortable, as there was no air-conditioning; they at least got you out of the sun. After a while a person stuck their head in and said, "Are there any women in here that would not mind talking to some reporters about what it's like to be a woman deployed?"

The media had centered its attention on the fact that this was the first major contingency where women were deploying in such large numbers. The United States had women deployed in past conflicts, but they did not receive the level of visibility as this deployment. I volunteered to speak with them, crawling out of the tent over to where I could sit on some pallets. They asked, "What is it like to deploy and did I have a husband or family that left back home?" I explained my husband was active duty and was actually getting ready to retire at the time after 20 years in the Air Force. Russ was extended on active duty due to the conflict but had not deployed. He was working and holding things together for our six-year-old daughter at home. Like all Air Force families, we had arrangements for child care and were committed to serve whether at home or deployed. I realized that it must seem difficult for those not serving in the military to understand the military mission and our commitment to serve. It is ingrained into our culture.

Military families, not just the active duty member, are committed to what is needed in a deployment. After this interview, a photo was taken and I went back to wait. It was not until months later that I would realize that my photo was released to the Associated Press nationwide. One of my best friends told me, "My mother in Wisconsin opened up the paper and about fell off the chair when she saw your picture." I was equally shocked. When I retired I was

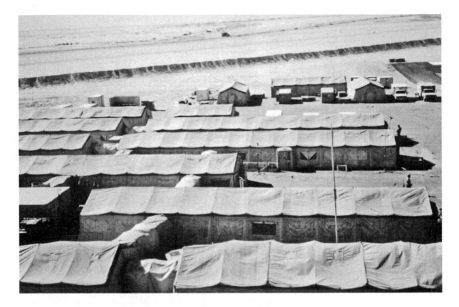

Tents have been a staple of United States military medicine for its entire history. The tent extendable modular personnel or TEMPER tent is used at military sites in the Persian Gulf Base of Operations. Constructed of vinyl coated duck cloth laid over a metal frame, the tent can be configured to any shape or size from a small personnel tent to a large hospital or cafeteria. It can be air-conditioned or heated, depending on the outside environment.

presented a paperback book which contained that photo. Life is full of surprises.

When I arrived at Thumrait, Oman, I met with the senior medical officer left in charge. As addressed earlier, our original hospital commander was sent home due to a medical condition. The next most senior officer was a psychiatrist. He had past deployment experience and did not hesitate stepping up to this position. There are a lot of posturing and emotions when people deploy, and it is critical that senior leaders pull together and have a united front in leading the troops. He asked for me to be his deputy commander and I welcomed the opportunity to serve in this position. Between the two of us we continued working plans to get the hospital operational.

Keep in mind that we were in a "secret location" in Oman. I am not sure as to why this location was not announced, as Oman has been one of the strongest supporters of U.S. presence in the Gulf since signing an access agreement with the U.S. in 1988. Oman supported the United States Air Force's prepositioned war reserve materiel (WRM). When I arrived I was amazed at what the wing had accomplished in the short time they had been there. They erected tent accommodations for base personnel and began work on establishing medical capabilities. The personnel arrived early August and the tent city was fully set up by September 15.

Setting up the hospital was a unique challenge. While we had pre–positioned ATH equipment and supplies, we did not have any tentage to build the hospital. We had to establish a way to provide medical care quickly, as personnel deploying into Oman included not only the 4th Wing assets but encompassed a composite wing which included Army aircraft along with Air Force and British aircraft, and this component was also growing. We were provided one half of an air-conditioned warehouse to set up a hospital. The other half was filled with MREs (meals ready to eat) and other war reserve material. Needless to say, that warehouse presented a number of challenges. It is amazing to think that a hardened facility would not be as good as a tent facility; but I have to say, we had it much better when we redeployed to Al-Kharj later and set up the ATH with our full component of tentage. We went back to the basics; completed an inventory of supplies, listed our requirements and began planning. We were cognizant of this massive movement of personnel across the theater, as well as in Europe, readying ourselves for the war. It was difficult to obtain additional supplies and equipment, so we resorted to building what we could.

The warehouse had one bathroom and the only sink in the warehouse was located in that one bathroom. How could we provide the privacy and care to our patients with thirty-foot ceilings, no walls, and florescent lighting? We had to figure out how we were going to accommodate the basic needs of these patients and how are we going to have sufficient lighting for these wards. We did not have any bedside commodes. So, we built bedside commodes. We only had cots that were very narrow and very difficult for patients to move on. When I got there the nurses didn't have any documentation forms and were spending hours taking pads of paper and making them look like the forms they needed. I told them to stop and we would move to narrative charting rather than creating our own forms. The availability of these simple tools would have made it so much easier for the personnel. On top of the pending threats and unknowns, we were forced to improvise and become innovative to meet basic needs.

Communication was critical. Rumors were rampant and could quickly destroy morale and discipline. To aid communication we took a wooden wall that we built to separate the hospital area in the warehouse from the supply end. This wall was lined with wide exam table paper, which was used to write the latest news. When you walked in to the hospital each day, you could immediately see the message board and know what was going on. This worked wonders in squelching many of the rumors. This sufficed, as e-mail was not available to us in the field. There were daily wing meetings to keep all the unit commanders abreast of latest development, as well as for us to report issues.

Pride in the uniform and professional appearance helped to maintain positive morale. Our wing commander said, "We may be here in the desert environment, but I will expect you to look sharp in your uniform, including your shoes, which will be appropriately maintained." This was a means to keep the troops focused, and it did boost morale and self–confidence. Even though we did not need people to work a six-day work week because we had plenty of staff, we maintained a six-day work week to limit free time. The base had limited facilities, and until we established recreational facilities, it proved advantageous to keep the unit working together. Personnel issues occupied our time, which included family problems, fear, and anxiety. We pulled together as a team and everyone watched out for each other.

Our hospital primarily cared for those that were injured at the base. We cared for deployed personnel that never should have been on mobility status because of pre–existing medical conditions, which included diabetics that were insulin dependent, severe chronic hypertension disease, etc. In a deployed environment with high temperatures, austere conditions, a stressful environment, and high physical demands, any chronic medical condition can be exacerbated. When you live and work in a close and contained area, there is a high risk for occupational injuries and accidents. While we did not treat war wounds, we had those that were injured locally. We did not know what to expect but planned for the worst case. We did perform elective surgeries in our mobile surgical unit as needed. We did not have the opportunity to arrange for medical care off the base.

One day we had an airman on base who worked with munitions disposal. While handling munitions, there was an explosion that resulted in a large portion of one of his hands being damaged. I witnessed staff that jumped right in delivering the emergency care, while there were others who responded appropriately but were visibly shaken up. This was one airman that was brought in with a blown up hand. As the chief nursing officer I questioned how to better prepare the personnel in dealing with what may come our way — more significant war injuries and deaths. We responded with more and more training. We did not have a lot of training materials with us, so we utilized the expertise of our medical staff and nurses.

In Oman we were so far removed from events in Iraq, I did not feel threatened by the pending war. The patient load was very light, and we established an aeromedical evacuation contingent. We heard that our air evaced ambulatory patients would be left at air bases within the theater to fend for themselves. They were being processed through the air evacuation system, but we were unable to communicate to their commanders in Oman as to their status. Again, we did not have any e-mail capability and phone service was very controlled. However, the military postal service (APO) was fairly reliable. In desperation, we started giving our patients self-addressed envelopes (mail service was free), so when they got to their respective locations, they could send notification back to us. This actually worked in many cases.

Morale would fluctuate widely, especially with each holiday. When November approached, we heard many of the hospital personnel saying, "We are going to be going home for Thanksgiving. Surely they are going to rotate us out. They are going to replace us and let us go home." There was a lot of that attitude, which was surprising to me because here we were readying ourselves for war; yet some thought we warranted a rotation. Why would anyone think that? Why would we rotate personnel out who have been acclimatized to the area and replace them with newly deployed troops? A big part of our job as leaders was to maintain high visibility with our personnel; listen to what they had to say, and keep their focus on the mission at hand. However, there was continued speculation that if we did not rotate in November, certainly it would occur by Christmas. I recalled the length of time troops deployed during our past two major conflicts—it could be years before we were sent home. Most did not want to even imagine that could occur.

Then we got the news. I looked upon it as the best news we could hear that would enable us to get over the holiday "hump." We were notified that we were re-deploying to Saudi Arabia. That gave everyone a brand-new focus. Instead of feeling morose about Christmas, everyone had to get into gear for this redeployment.

Our 4th Medical Group wing commander, Colonel Hal Hornburg, who ran the composite forces at Thumrait would continue to be the composite wing commander at Al-Kharj. He allowed us to transport not only what we needed from our Thumrait location, but those comfort items we had accumulated. Therefore, we were not limited by Typical bathroom tent just what we could carry with us in our mobility bags, but what could be transported on pallets. This helped lift the morale of the troops during this transition.

Colonel Hornberg was a visible leader that made a point to visit the different base units. As members of the wing were admitted to the hospital, he would take the time to visit them and speak words of encouragement. He had high expectations of performance for all that served in the wing; and all had a great deal of respect for his leadership. He had a mission to complete and we were kept informed of the expectations and the challenges. His confidence increased confidence in others, and we were clear on what we needed to accomplish. He was decisive, but yet did not keep isolated from his troops. When we celebrated Christmas prior to leaving Thumrait, his wife sent him a camouflaged Santa outfit that he wore to the Christmas celebrations. It was nice to see the human side of our leaders.

The new location was located in the desert — in the middle of nowhere — and came to be known as "Al-Kharj," or "Al's Garage," during Operations Desert Shield and Storm (currently called Prince Sultan Air Base). It was

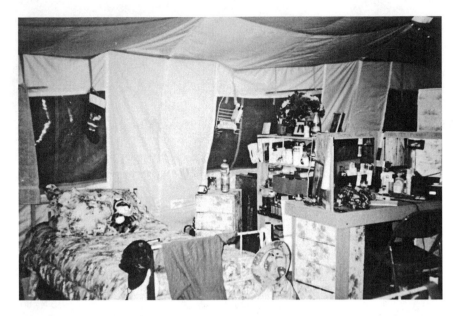

Senior officer tents housed four occupants with vanities built by base civil engineers.

located 60 miles south of Riyadh. It had an immense 15,000-foot runway with a parking area, and little else. During Desert Shield, the coalition forces built Al-Kharj from scratch. From October 1990 to March 1991, a combined 435-person RED HORSE squadron was involved in more than 25 major projects, valued at more than $14.6 million. These projects included bedding down the largest air base in theater (in terms of number of aircraft — capable of bedding down five fighter squadrons) at Al-Kharj Air Base. Seventeen K-span facilities were built and roads carved out. RED HORSE, augmented by the 4th CES from Seymour Johnson AFB, NC, and contract personnel, hauled 200,000 cubic yards of clay to build a foot-thick clay foundation for our tent city. Eventually, an entire tent city was established which included four kitchens, our 50-bed air transportable hospital, six K-span structures, and support facilities. They built munitions storage areas and bladder berms, completed utility distribution systems, and installed mobile aircraft arresting systems. In less than two months in 1990, Al-Kharj changed from a base without buildings and only a ramp and runways, to a base with dining halls, hangars, a hospital, electric power generators, and services for an expanded population of Air Force personnel. Al-Kharj was ready for aircraft early in January 1991, and by the beginning of the war was home to 4,900 Air Force personnel.

Even though we were in the middle of the desert, the new base was set up in a highly organized fashion with security and privacy as key considerations. They had established high berms that provided a natural perimeter around our base. We were told the base would expand quickly and it did. As stated previously, we ended up with over 5,000 people on our base. Our tent city was separate from where the operational flight line was located. Again, this supported security but also made it quieter in the living area and where the hospital was located. Scud missiles were a concern, and you just hoped that perhaps the military targets such as the aircraft or flight line would be targeted rather than the tent city. I certainly was not aware of the accuracy of these missiles, but you rationalize such things to allay your fears.

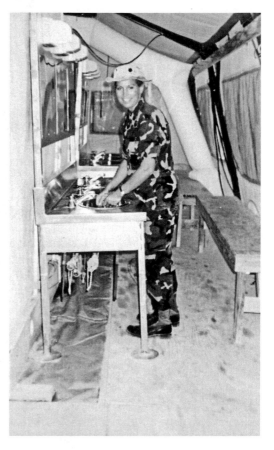

Jane Valentine cleaning up in the community female toilet facility.

Our new tent city design at Al-Kharj was much improved to Thumrait. But then we did not have to build it around other base structures but had an empty slate upon which to set the design. In Thumrait the shower tents were located in the midst of the general living tentage areas. Also, the male and female tents were located fairly close together, and we had experienced a couple instances of peeping toms. Even though the shower and toilet facilities were in marked tents, separate for women and men, we had situations where people stated that they did not know which was which. Steps were taken to provide a much safer environment. The Al-Kharj tent city had all the women tentage located down the first two rows of tent city with their shower and bathroom facilities located at a completely separate location from the men. The men had another 30 or more rows of tents. There was no way that there could be any confusion, absolutely no reason why any man should be around our bathroom facilities (or vice versa).

Most of the tents were eight to ten people, but as a senior officer I was placed in a tent with another field grade officer who was the JAG or Judge Advocate General. Both of our husbands were Air Force officers who were not deployed and generously ensured that we had all the comforts of home. Between the two spouses, we were set up with a microwave, bed comforters, portable closets, refrigerator, and bicycles. Others also had comfort items sent to them. We either had them sent on pallets from Seymour Johnson Air Base, if there was extra room available, or they were mailed. This was a key morale booster.

Al-Kharj was built with more permanent structures, including paved roads. All of our tents had electricity and air-conditioning. We had everything we needed to operate efficiently and effectively. There were vehicles provided to those that required them; however, women were not allowed to drive off base. If we needed to go into town, we had the support of male drivers. Most of us walked everywhere, and I had my bike. We did have a brief problem with the men "cruising" in their vehicles up and down the female tent rows. I am sure they enjoyed viewing the girls taking advantage of sun bathing next to their tents. But we quickly put a stop to that with establishing a "no cruising" rule. We tried our best to maintain privacy in such close and restricted quarters. Men and women could visit in each others' tents, but there had to be agreement of your tentmates to have such visitors. Of course, no overnight visitation.

General Norman Schwarzkopf issued General Order #1 which did not allow any use of alcohol. In Oman alcohol was not restricted by the Oman people, and therefore it was allowed on base until General Order #1 was issued. This alcohol restriction was a very positive move, as there were a number of alcohol-related incidents that we dealt with prior to the restriction. It is best not to allow drinking in the deployed environment if it cannot be controlled somehow.

As I have mentioned, the new challenge in Saudi Arabia were the Scud missile alerts. Scud missiles are mobile, Russian-made, short-range, tactical ballistic surface-to-surface missiles. Now that we were further north in Saudi Arabia, we were possibly in range of the Scud missiles. Still I found solace in the fact that we were not as close as many of the other Air Force bases in theater. I attended an in-theater Air Force deployed ATH chief nurse's conference at one location where they had Patriot missile batteries located right outside of the perimeter fence in easy view. These Patriot missiles are used to destroy the Scud missiles before they reach their intended location. Therefore, this particular base was at a much higher risk for Scud attacks. The chief nurses' meeting was an excellent opportunity for us to discuss lessons learned and many deployment issues and challenges.

At Al-Kharj, despite our location, we had many Scud alerts which required donning chemical warfare gear, including gas masks, and seeking

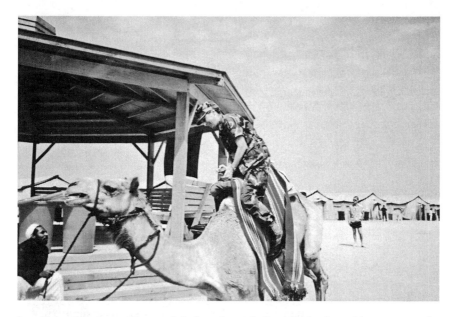

Jane Valentine sits on the camel the base brought in as method to raise troop morale. This gave base personnel the opportunity to sit for a photo and take a ride around the gazebo.

cover in the bunkers. As a result of the impaired vision from the masks, we had several serious injuries when airmen tripped over tent lines and other obstructions.

At Al-Kharj our ATH was brand new and included full tentage and supplies. We all participated in setting up the structure once the blacktop or asphalt was installed. This asphalt surfacing was a blessing, as we experienced rainy periods in the desert that created beds of mud. We also built a helipad near the hospital, which was used periodically. The ATH were located approximately one-fourth mile or less from the tent city and several miles from where the aircraft were located. The tent doorway zippers do not last very long on these tents; and the base civil engineers helped by building wooden doors. These were very functional and many personalized their doors. There was a lot of creativity seen throughout tent city with these doors. It brought the tent mates together with camaraderie and provided a bit of levity in a very serious environment. We grew to a population of 5,000. We, therefore, had a reasonably high census in our hospital. We had full dental services, operating rooms, two inpatient wards and outpatient services. Our base was self-contained and our nurses were busy.

Our civil engineering personnel, or the RED HORSE team, had extra wood after building base structures and built wooden floors in our personnel's

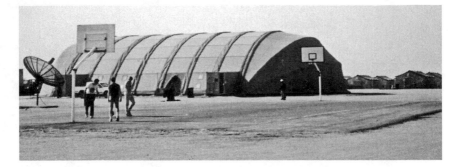

Deployed troops took advantage of base facilities to improve overall fitness and divert their attention from the extended deployment and risks. The base gymnasium was complete with a weight room donated by Arnold Schwarzenegger.

tents — a little more touch of comfort. Arnold Schwartzenegger donated complete gym equipment to Al-Kharj to set up a huge gym for base personnel. Our base CE (civil engineering) personnel built mirrors inside the gym, and with the extra mirrors they hand built vanities for each of the female tents. I was moved by their thoughtfulness, and the women enjoyed the luxury of having a piece of "furniture" in their tents. In Al-Kharj we still had eight to ten people in tents, so you did not have that much privacy, but we provided more permanent beds — old Russian metal beds. It is certainly proven that there is a lot less trouble with one's mental and physical status if you reside in a safe environment that provides a decent place to sleep.

I thought of our time in Thumrait; when we had Army air units co-located with us. Some of them expressed that the Air Force personnel were "soft." I did not see that we were soft, but we took the opportunity to improve the quality of life for our troops. Not that the Army does not try to achieve this as well. I feel that the Air Force had less numbers to provide for, and therefore, the capability to provide more. Also, we were not as mobile and our hospitals were not located on the front lines. We did what we could to provide a bit of privacy and comforts if available. Air force or Army — all U.S. military forces had highly qualified combatants and healthcare providers.

We took care of our patients in the desert as we did at home. One thing I remembered was the challenge of the Scud alerts and getting the patients out of the hospital into the bunker next to the hospital. Not all the patients could be removed from their equipment and taken to the bunkers. We evacuated those patients that could be moved to the hospital bunker, but there were others that had to be left behind. The nurses stayed with their patients, protecting them as they could be with padding and assisting them with their gas masks. All alerts were considered to be real Scud attacks; therefore, these nurses and technicians were risking their lives for their patients.

Everyone had their own way to cope with the stress. Many rationalized in their own minds that they were beyond Scud range. They had faith that the Patriot missiles would protect us. We had the high berms built around the base and you relied on the base security to prevent any infiltration into the base, but you never knew for sure. We were always vigilant, always on high alert while there. We all pulled together and worked together, supporting each other.

There were many challenges to leadership. We had anonymous notes left for the commander. One day a scorpion was left on his desk in a glass jar with a note stating, "We feel as trapped as this bug in the jar, and we know you're the one holding us here." Some were convinced that they had an opportunity to go home but leadership chose to have us stay. We had to work through those things, and we did successfully. Nothing ever deteriorated to the point where it started breaking down the organization.

Desert Storm began January 17. I remember distinctly hearing our aircraft taking off. I said a prayer for their safe return. We had all come to know many of the crew, and once again another sense of reality set in. We could have some of our friends and colleagues not return.

I tried not to let the risks of our deployment impact me personally— tried to remain upbeat and positive. One time I had a challenge when I received orders to select a number of our hospital personnel to be deployed to a forward location in support of a chemical recovery team. I thought that I could be selecting individuals for harm's way. I did not hesitate in complying with such orders; but I complied with thinking of each person as an individual and what impact that could have on them and their families. I wished them well as they moved on. They all redeployed home at the war's end, safe and sound.

Al-Kharj became a showcase of sorts. We had foreign military personnel who were very impressed with what we had accomplished, and medical teams that found our air transportable hospital amazing. We therefore were very much involved in public relations, in demonstrating our capabilities to our host allies. We became familiarized with different cultural requirements and were respectful of these.

So what of the medical care we provided? I would say that whether you are in a base hospital in North Carolina or you are caring for a patient in a tent, patient care is still patient care. That came naturally to all of us at our deployed location. While in Thumrait, we were under a water restriction and had only a single bathroom in our warehouse hospital. We had to work within severe constraints and we did so successfully. However, the normal environmental maintenance and cleanliness we had stateside was no longer available to us. We learned to work within these constraints and prioritized as to what we could get accomplished with what we had. When we moved to Saudi Arabia and were able to set up a full air transportable hospital, we had everything we needed. We did not have a bathroom on each ward or a sink at each bed, but we learned to function.

I wrote in my deployment notes that in some instances we had more at Al-Kharj than we had at home in the States. At the time when I deployed, I had been trying to get a personal computer for my office. Back in those years, personal computers were not as available to all staff as they are today. My administrative assistant had a computer, but I was having difficulty gaining the authorization for a computer for myself. The commander prioritized what offices got computers, such as finance and supply departments. When we were in Saudi Arabia, we had computers at all of our desks. It is interesting to realize that my beginning reliance on a PC started with my deployment to the Gulf War!

Communication was a challenge of a different sort when we moved up to Saudi Arabia. Not that we lacked means for communication, but open access to telephones offered additional challenges. AT&T provided several phones for troops to use right within our hospital as well in a central location at the base. This allowed families close contacts with their loved ones that were deployed. While you would think this would be positive, it also placed a lot of pressure on our troops. Personal issues at home crept into the deployed work place. Accusations of affairs and improprieties and family problems caused morale problems. Therefore, sometimes there can be too much communication. As I addressed previously, this was quite different from when we were at Thumrait, where we relied on exam paper with the latest news; and the occasional letter from home. At Al-Kharj we heard of all the political news going on at home along with the personal issues at home, over both of which we had little control and had to keep on top of maintaining morale. It could easily distract attention from getting the job done at hand.

Deployments taxed relationships that were not strong. Any type of conflict can easily tear a person apart; especially when they are helpless in being able to resolve the issue while deployed. Staff did not know what the near future would hold. Would we stay at Al-Kharj? How long would the war last? When would we go home? We did not know what was going to happen next. As leaders, we constantly worked hard to maintain a cohesive team. But a conflict at home, unsubstantiated rumors, the unknown, all can be challenging. These we faced and these we were able to overcome amongst the staff. For me, I did not have any personal issues to resolve. I was fortunate to have a wonderful husband who managed our daughter and understood I had a job to do. Therefore, I was able to concentrate my efforts on the job to be done. Others did not have that support, and it showed.

Another means of communication we had was our base public address system which was also called the "giant voice." Many referred to it as the "giant whisper" because many times we had difficult hearing it due to malfunctions.

Sometimes it would blast the message, other times you could not hear it at portions of the base or it would fade in and out. Technology was not always desert tolerant.

Another item that I recall being difficult involved our contracted employees that provided us laundry and food services support. While at Thumrait, we took care of our own services, including washing our clothes by hand in large trash cans. It was very antiquated but it actually provided a means to pass the time on your day off. When we moved to Saudi, we were much busier with patient care and the base was much larger, making it more difficult to maintain. The base therefore utilized contracted foreign workers.

All of us had our chemical warfare gear for when there were Scud alerts. When we had our first couple of Scud alerts, we donned our chemical protective gear as trained. The giant voice alerted us to Scud alerts and would announce the MOPP status, or what level of protective gear had to be donned. As I donned my gear, I observed the service workers putting plastic bags over their heads as some means of protection. It was disheartening. However, not long after that these first few alerts, the contract workers were at least provided respirator devices. Some worried about these contract workers sabotaging us. Fortunately, I did not have this fear and trusted the screening process that was used to hire them on.

It was very unfortunate that we experienced several personal casualties. While building Al-Kharj, we lost an airman that was killed during the construction. I am not aware of the details, but the wing stenciled "not one more life" all over the base after his death to maintain a heightened awareness for safety. As for direct war related incidents, we did have one of our pilots captured when his plane was shot down and he was confined as a POW for a while. We also lost a crew when another F-15E was shot down. That pilot was unique as he was also one of our flight surgeons that worked at our hospital. Each day as our planes took off, I wondered if they would all return.

Did we feel at risk? I cannot speak for others, but the alerts to the bunkers and donning the chemical gear was a bit harrowing. We would be alerted at all hours of the night. As we fell into the bunkers built near our tents, I would look around and would wonder if what I was seeing in the dark night was a vapor or was it just the obstructed vision of the mask. I would wonder when we would have injuries or symptoms displayed from a gas attack. But then we would hear the "all clear," and relief would set in and I realized that all was fine once again. In some ways you do get somewhat used to all of this. You respond as you have trained, always thinking, "Thank God, that wasn't anything," and continue working or return to your tents to sleep. The body and the mind adapt to these things—for some better than others.

I was very much attuned to the cultural differences that were imposed in both Oman and Saudi Arabia. This was a unique war environment due to

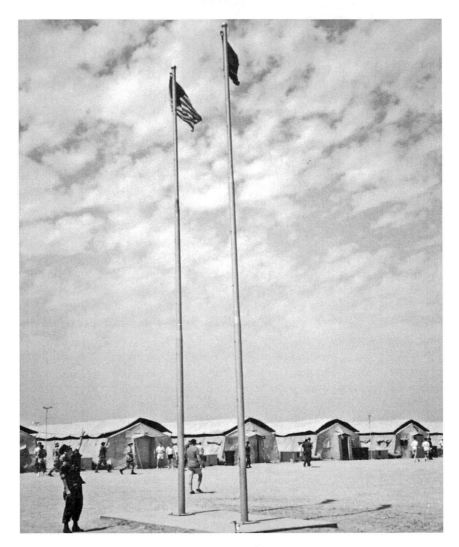

It was an honor to have our flag displayed. After waiting months to have military legal negotiate terms for us to be able to raise the American flag at the base, Jane Valentine points proudly at the stars and stripes.

the number of women who deployed and the requirements the women had to comply with if we departed the base. I felt fortunate that we had the freedom we did on our base, as our isolated location allowed us to wear what we wanted off duty (i.e., shorts and T-shirts); while others that were located nearer to the local communities had stricter dress codes, especially if they were in visible sight of the nationals.

There was one restriction that I did resent strongly — we were not allowed to fly the American Flag over our base. I have always had a great love for our flag and the pride in my country that it represented. I also thought of those that had died and risked their lives to fight a war in this theater; and yet we could not serve under our flag. Our wing lawyers worked diligently on this restriction until an agreement was finally met. When the agreement was signed, a large flag pole was placed in the middle of the base's common center of tent city and the flag was raised. That meant a lot for all of us. This was one of the more emotional events for me during the deployment — when they raised the flag that day. The flag pole stood in a central location of tent city that we called the "mall." This area contained many of the services needed such as a post office, church, small store, a bank of AT&T phones, a gazebo and other service buildings or tents. Our flag flying overhead certainly fanned the patriotism in all of us. I felt honored to have this opportunity to serve my country.

When I heard that the war was over, I wondered if it really was. Were we really going home? We were so excited; what a rush of emotions and feelings. The number one thought was finally returning home to our families. The next was feeling relief for our safety and the safety of our air crews. It was an unbelievable feeling — hard to describe. Finally hearing what I dreamed about for months was going to happen. As reality set in, we planned our departure. We left most everything at the base as more reserve units were going to come in to replace us. I left many of the comfort items that I had accumulated, including my bike, refrigerator, bedding, etc. This was very appreciated by our replacements. Eventually hardened buildings replaced the tent city, and Al-Kharj became a permanent base.

As deployed troops returning home, we met an outpouring of support and praise. I flew home on a military transport flight with my unit and had a very emotional stop in Suffrage, New Hampshire. I was overwhelmed with patriotism of this town. Once we landed, base personnel informed us: "We have some people from the community that really want to show their appreciation for your service in the Gulf. We want to prepare you for when you go into that hanger as there are a lot of people there." You would not believe what then happened. There were thousands of people waiting for us— we were not their sons or daughters— but strangers that they came to welcome. They praised us as heroes. I did not think of myself as a hero, but someone who did what we were trained and committed to do. I thought back to the Vietnam War and how terribly the returning troops were treated. I was overwhelmed with emotion, with pride and honor.

Once I returned home, certainly I came across individuals that were critical of our country's decision to embark on this conflict. But usually I found these individuals had no concept of the volunteer force and that we chose to join the military. Most were individuals who never served in the military and could not understand. As members of an all-volunteer force, we had full understanding of the possibility of serving in a conflict or war. We trained for this continuously while serving in our peacetime roles.

Family was so very important to me throughout my deployment. My husband was "one in a million" and was the strength for me and our daughter, Ashley. She was just six years old and starting first grade when I deployed. Ashley suffered nightmares while I was gone because of all the war scenes she saw on television. Russ kept her very busy, wrapping packages daily to send to mom, cooking and creating pictures, paintings and all kinds of projects. He took photos constantly of the two of them, and every couple of weeks I would receive a new photo book complete with captioned photos of all of their activities together. Despite him working full time, he made every time they were together a special event. They cooked together, shopped, created pictures and planned activities. He was so successful in keeping her mind off of the war and keeping me in touch with them. I do not believe if our roles were switched, that I could have done all that my husband did. This was a unique bonding experiencing for the two of them, which could never be matched. I believe Ashley grew up to be such a strong, giving, trusting and beautiful woman as a result of my husband's love and dedication to family.

There was quite a bit of press that addressed the fact that this war differed from previous ones due to the number of women that deployed. There were families that had extreme difficulties with this. In my family we were both active duty and experienced a number of separations prior to this extended deployment. Perhaps these separations strengthened our relationships and enabled us to deal with the deployment as we did. From the start of our marriage, the Air Force challenged us with separations. After our marriage while in Germany, Russ returned stateside prior to me. Before I relocated to Seymour Johnson, Russ had already transferred to North Carolina 18 months prior to us gaining a joint spouse assignment. Even when we were stationed together, his job as a pilot had him gone for days at a time. Of course all of these separations do not compare with a deployment, but it certainly built a strong relationship that enabled us to cope.

Once I returned from the deployment, it was a bit hard adjusting to a more normal life-style. Deployment is a very physical and mental experience. As a result, I delved into a number of activities that I probably would have never ventured into if it was not for the deployment. Looking back, over the time while deployed, I had built a sense of invincibility. One becomes mentally and physically focused on survival. During my deployment I met a cadre of friends who were dedicated sky divers. Over the months of talking of home and what we planned when we returned, skydiving became part of my list of "to dos." One of my roommates, the lawyer, and I planned to do this together with our husbands. Upon our return, both our spouses were not happy with this plan at all. The old adage "Why jump out of a perfectly good airplane?" was stated more than once. Therefore, I decided to schedule my sky dive when my husband was out of town on a trip so he wouldn't worry so much. I was heading out for my big day, when he called to inform me he was home early. I admitted to him my plans, and without hesitation he came out to join me. Russ is certainly not a risk taker, but he did want to be with me and took the leap. This was no easy feat, as we had to climb out onto the landing gear of a flying Cessna at 10,000 feet with the tandem dive instructor strapped with a four-point strap to your back. Russ went first, but my jump was not without incident. Once he landed and as he looked up at the sky, he asked his instructor if I had a starter chute that would be released first. He was quickly informed that it appeared that my first chute failed to deploy and was released, but not to be concerned, as the tandem instructor also had a chute. Fortunately, it deployed without a problem. Even better — I had no idea there was a problem until I had two feet on the ground.

While deployed, I took advantage of running — and did a lot of running; sometimes morning and evening. I had a sense of freedom when I ran. It was such a relief to get out of the heavy combat boots and fatigues, put on shorts and a T-shirt, and run the tent perimeter. It cleared my head and restored my soul in a way. Upon my return, I decided to train further and run the Sixteenth Annual Marine Corps Marathon held in Washington D.C. on November 3, 1991. Despite Russ hating to run, he trained with me. I think we had been separated so long that we did not want to be apart — even while training for this event. He was the best! It can get very hot in North Carolina in the late summer and early fall. Before we would start running our ten miles, Russ would drive out first and pre–position water bottle along the side of the road every three miles so we could get water and would not become dehydrated. He finished the 26 miles and 385 yards in 4 hours and 39 minutes, and I trailed behind in at 4 hours and 51 minutes. It was amazing.

Before leaving Seymour Johnson AFB, I also had the opportunity to fly in the back seat of an F-15 Eagle. With the aircraft's large canopy, you felt like to you were sitting on the outside of the plane. It was one of the most exciting events of my life.

Russ soon retired from the Air Force and was flying for United Parcel Service. We not only had to adjust to a renewed life together, he was embarking on a second career. Fortunately, it was one that a PCS move would not interfere with him getting to work as long as there was a major airport close by. UPS has him flying a week and home a week; therefore, I was back into a pseudo single-parenting role for myself, as Russ was gone at least 50 percent of the time. But we pulled together as a family and endured as always.

Jane went on to serve at Langley Air Force Base, at Maxwell Air Force Base as chief nurse, and at MacDill Air Force Base as medical support squadron com-

mander and chief nurse. She retired in 2000 and in 2001 became corporate director of patient care services for Shriner's Hospitals for Children. In her summary of her military career she says:

Nursing was my professional calling. Service in the Air Force provided me the professional growth and opportunity to serve that is unequaled in any other avenue. I must say how very fortunate I was to have had the experience I did in their force and deployment to Desert Shield/Desert Storm. It was an interesting seven months deployment full of planning, innovations, flexibility, hard work, camaraderie, professional growth and pride.

When I was in the Air Force, there were many who did not plan for deployment and had a difficult time facing it when it occurred. I witnessed a number of reservists who actually said, "I did not join the reserves to be put on active duty." Fortunately, the majority felt this was their duty that they were committed to it.

Troops today understand that they are part of an all-volunteer force. It is very clear today that when you join the military, you will be deployed and with deployments you place your life on the line. I wish the media would display this side — the true side of troops' resolve to serve the mission. The American people need to understand that, accept that, support our commander-in-chief, and support the troops.

CAROL WHITESIDES

Nurses are amazing men and women with brilliant minds and the ability to apply their knowledge in new and creative ways. Carol Whitesides has a bachelor's degree in microbiology and chemistry, worked in biologic research during the Vietnam era, and has a bachelor's degree in nursing. She received a master's degree in public administration and health science from the Marriott Center of Management in the Marriot Business School at Brigham Young University (BYU), one of the highest ranked business schools in the United States. She assisted in designing a children's hospital and became the director of surgical services at that hospital.

At the age of 42 she joined the United States Navy Nurse Corps reserves and went back to get a second master's degree as a family nurse practitioner (FNP). She says, "I wanted something that I could work at when I got older. I love nursing. I want to continue practicing nursing." She experienced two tours of service during the Persian Gulf Wars, adapting to two different types of environments. After her active duty military experience, she went on to assist in world humanitarian efforts.

When I graduated in the early '90s from BYU, I went to work as a nurse practitioner for the Navy. One of the Navy docs I was with in reserves asked me to come and practice with him up in Layton, Utah, in a family practice clinic. I joined their family practice group.

Before I got my FNP I was called up for Desert Storm. We knew something was happening because they started getting us prepped at the reserve center. The whole unit was called up. They all went to Saudi except me. I wasn't called up. I was really kind of disappointed and wondered what was going on. A week or two later I was called up individually to Adak, Alaska. I asked, "Why Adak?" They told me all the nurses stationed at Adak were taken and there were none up there. I said, "First of all, where is Adak?" When we were called up to Desert Storm, we didn't go according to our NOBC or designator number. Mine was in the operating room. They put people who had never been in the operating room before into the operating room.

I flew to San Francisco and up to Elmendorf, Alaska. I stayed overnight and got on a plane transport to Adak. Adak is eight hours out to the end of the Aleutian chain. It's the second island from the end of the Aleutian chain.

At that time Adak had a nuclear weapon on the island, and we went because the Marines were there. I was an operating room nurse. I hadn't worked the floors as a staff nurse for many years. I ended up being the only nurse in a 15 bed hospital. This island was interesting because they had the Marines and their families. P-3 pilots flew in monitoring subs going through the straits from Russia. The island had been occupied by the Japanese during World War II. Before you could leave the airport, you were issued a parka and survival gear for the weather. I was issued an old Army green 1950s car.

It was lovely when I got there. I never did see the sun because the mist was in all the time. You weren't allowed to go off any roadway more than 50 feet because the Japanese had put pongee spikes and other booby traps all over the island. If you were to go hiking, you must be escorted by someone who knew the trails. Because of the location the temperature could drop and it could get very nasty. The rain is kind of sleety rain all the time. You couldn't go off on your own unless you had special training in cold weather survival. The base did not take up the whole island. We had about ten miles of road and of that only five were paved. The other thing that was interesting was the puffins and the bald eagles.

There were no other inhabitants on the island except the Marines and their families. There was no town. The BOQ was interesting. The windows would not open because of the weather, the doors wouldn't stay closed. The P-3 pilots would walk by and wave at any time of the day or night. It was always daylight because it was summer. If you wanted to sleep you had to put your blanket up on the window because there was no drapery. We had no television except for one military channel. In the 15 bed hospital you didn't have a kitchen, and so I would have to send a corpsman to the mess hall for the patients' dinners.

The hospital was 15 individual rooms. The first patient I had was a mother who had strep and the baby was septic. We had a number of military psych problems. The only doctor was a brand new doctor who had just finished his residency. He was a pediatrician. That was good because he could help with the baby. But from then on he just didn't know what to do. We had an attempted suicide, alcohol intoxication, gastritis and any number of different medical problems. When patients came in drunk, we would have one of their buddies come and watch them. Then they would have to clean the ward the next morning.

The most interesting patient there was a fisherman who had fallen down into the bottom of his boat. He had a flail chest. They were not going to let him come onto island because he wasn't military. Finally, they said he could come and wait until he could be transported off. We had to intubate and bag him, and it took eight hours for a plane to pick him up.

My biggest problem was scrounging for food. The supply barge would come in on Thursday with fresh food, and so you'd have to rush down to the exchange to buy your food, otherwise you'd get dinners that were two or three years outdated. I had a fridge in the room and a microwave in the hall. They didn't have an officer's club. Once in a while I'd go down to the NCO club but they didn't have fresh food either. Desert Storm was so short, and since I didn't get called up until the shooting started, I wasn't in Adak very long. I was there about four weeks.

I was pretty lucky compared to some of the others in our unit who went to the Gulf. One of our nurses stepped off a bus and tripped over her gas mask and broke her nose. Another got a horrible sinus infection from the blowing wind. Just recently an Army nurse I knew who had been called up to Saudi died of leukemia.

I didn't have a whole lot of information about what was going on with the war. I didn't have much notice about coming home, only about 48 hours. I did get an offer from the P-3 pilots to ride from Adak down to the Easter or Canary Islands, but I never did do that. I did get to see one video show. One night a ship came in from NOAA, the weather people. They would let them dock, but they were not allowed get off their boat. I went down to talk with them, and they invited me back that night for pizza and videos. I didn't get to see much of Alaska. I flew directly into Adak and out again. It was such a short war.

I came back to work, and shortly after finished school, I went to work full time as a nurse practitioner and part-time teaching at Weber State. I stayed in the Navy. My husband took early retirement and we moved to Las Vegas. I took a job with the VA at the federal hospital on Nellis Air Force Base. Three months into that job I was recalled to the second war. The reserve unit in Vegas was part of Camp Pendleton. We had spent several summers training at Camp Pendleton. We would do two weeks of fleet hospital training. For fleet hospital training we would be put in a confined area. They locked us in this high barbwire fence about a mile square where we lived in fleet hospital conditions. The Marines would come by with their helicopters and shoot smoke bombs over our heads and would try to penetrate our parameters. I was also sent to the Army's combat casualty course.

Our unit had no idea what was happening at the beginning of the second war. Some of the corpsmen in our unit had been called up, so we knew it was in the wind. I got a call on a Friday afternoon to report Monday morning in San Diego. I was just getting ready to go home from work. It was 3:30 in the afternoon. I called personnel letting them know I would not be to work on Monday.

It took two weeks to process us, which was different from the first war where it took about three days. I didn't have my orders so I didn't know where I was going to be sent. I did go to Camp Pendleton and worked for about a year in the internal medicine clinic. I lived in the BOQ right by the beach.

While at Camp Pendleton I work in the internal medical clinic during the day but three evenings a week we received wounded. The military had the philosophy of sending their wounded back to their stations instead of to a general medical facility. So if the Marine was from Camp Pendleton, they would go from Germany to Andrews Air force base and be dispersed as quickly as possible across the United States back to their station areas. I disagree with this for two reasons. It was harder to keep count of exactly how many were wounded, which I think was part of the rational of doing it. Some of wounded would move so quickly that we received them after they had traveled for 24 hours without pain medications. They would also be two or three days without their malaria medication. There was some disconnect in treating the troops from the time they left Germany to arriving at their home stations because they had been dispersed so quickly. Of course the real serious ones they would keep. It was sad seeing these 21-year-old Marines with their hands blown off or blind or with severe head injuries, and they had wife with a baby they'd never seen. That was the hard part of the war. The Marines, no matter how badly they were hurt, were ready to go back and fight some more. They didn't want to be taken out of service.

In the evening I would do the family practice walk-in clinic for children and families. I worked eight hours in the clinic and then about five hours in the evening every day. I had Saturdays and Sundays off. These hours weren't bad. It wasn't physically hard. You'd get off in the evening and walk on the beach.

It was March of 2003 when I got to San Diego, and I was on active duty there until 2004. Towards the end of the war something happened with the Navy, BUMED and the Pentagon. They seemed to have some kind of disagreement. All of a sudden the Navy said we were all going home. Within 24 hours all active reservists were discharged. Camp Pendleton learned the Navy would not be sending any replacements. Doctor Petell, the commander over the clinic, was really upset. He did not want me to leave. He said, "You can't just leave." He called BUMED and said, "We need these people. We need to leave them here. They can't so home yet." He was told we were to be out in 24 hours, and we were gone.

There were so many people sent to San Diego for discharge they couldn't process us out fast enough. Many of us were sent to Bremerton for discharge. I was fine with going to Bremerton. It took two weeks to process us for discharge. It was like another two-week paid vacation. I then came back home and settled into my job and reserve status. Shortly after returning home I got a call from BUMED letting me know they were getting my papers ready again. This time I would be an OR nurse in Iraq. There was only one problem. I was

60 years old. They wanted me to please sign the age waiver they were sending. I said, "I don't think so." They sent the waiver anyway.

I wouldn't have minded going back to California and Camp Pendleton or doing other nurse practitioner jobs, but they were getting my OR NOBC ready, and I knew I would be in Iraq in tents and in fleet-type positions. The Navy was using the Army field hospitals in Iraq because the foot print of our fleet hospital was too big. They were integrating into the Army hospitals. The other thing they were doing was sending the Air Force out to Afghanistan over and over. They were also sending small surgical contingency groups out. They called them FASS deployed units. They were sending some of the Navy people with them. This would have been a lot of physical labor and at 60 years old, I didn't think I could do the desert and live in tents. Personnel were being sent to the desert for 15 months at this time. I didn't want to experience those living in those conditions at my age . At 60 your joints don't work as well, especially in those harsh conditions. If they had sent me back down to Pendleton and I worked 16 hours a day doing office practice, I could have done that. I can live in fairly harsh conditions, but not for 15 months. I only had 16 years in, and I would have had to sign a waiver for every year after 60 in order to get my 20 years. Since I did not sign the age waiver, I was discharged from the service.

I stayed in Vegas after I returned from my active duty. I went to work as a nursing administrator at one of the hospitals. I stayed in Vegas for a couple of years and then moved back to Utah to care for elderly parents. I'm currently working part time as a nurse practitioner and full time as a teacher at Salt Lake Community College. Salt Lake Community College sent me to Shanghai, China, to teach for six weeks. Last year I went to Mali, Africa, on a medical mission for Mali Rising Foundation. I worked as a NP seeing about 100 patients a day. We also saw whatever happened to come through the door. The Mali Rising Foundation wants me to set up another trip for Africa this year. I'm working with some of the OB-GYN physicians from Salt Lake and Ogden. We meet once a month and talk about setting up clinics for training African nurses to do health care. It's not just about flying in there and helping the people and flying out. We also try to make a lasting impression on the people.

REFERENCES

Cullpepper, M., and P. Adams, 1988. Nursing in the Civil War. *American Journal of Nursing:* 981–984.

Helmstadter, C. 2003. A real tone: professionalizing nursing in nineteenth-century London. *Nursing History Review* 11: 3–30.

Nurses at War. Nurses at war project. http://nursing.byu.edu/nursesatwar/.

Prince Sultan Air Base, Al-Kharj, Saudi Arabia. http://www.globalsecurity.org/military/facility/prince-sultan.htm

Purcell, M. 2000. District #9 Civil War nursing conference winning essay: Angels of mercy. *District News:* 18–19.

Rogge, M. M. 1987. Nursing and politics: A forgotten legacy. *Nursing Research* 36(1).

Rushton, P., L. Callister, & M. Wilson, 2005. *Latter-day Saint nurses at war: A story of caring and sacrifice.* Prove: Religious Studies, Brigham Young University.

INDEX